Praise for *The Intimate Herbal*

"As a woman who went through a lot of hormonal turmoil in my thirties, I know firsthand how using herbs and plant wisdom can bring us back to balance. I am so grateful for herbalists and writers like Marie White who are guiding us toward these beautiful, nourishing ways."

—SHIVA ROSE, author of *Whole Beauty*, alchemist, mama, and creator of Shiva Rose Beauty

"*The Intimate Herbal* is as practical as it is inspiring. Complete with herbal foundations for people of all levels of experience as well as comprehensive, holistic approaches to preventative care, imbalances, and herbal therapeutics, it creates a pathway into self-determined healing that is at once important to both the individual and the collective. People of all genders can find within these pages the tools for healing, pleasure, and renewal."

—BRITTANY WOOD NICKERSON, founder of Thyme Herbal and author of *Recipes from the Herbalist's Kitchen* and *The Herbal Homestead Journal*

"*The Intimate Herbal* is a powerful contribution to the literature available on sexual and reproductive health. Marie's herbal knowledge shines through on every page as she skillfully weaves together information from the latest scientific research and her own practice. Her clear explanations about herbal terminology and preparations as well as her specific recipes make this book both useful and empowering. It's a treasure trove of herbal goodness for anyone seeking sexual vitality!"

—KIMBERLY GALLAGHER, author of *Aphrodisiac*, cofounder of LearningHerbs, and creator of Wildcraft!

"*The Intimate Herbal* is a wonderful demonstration of what it can look like to thrive as a grassroots herbalist in a modern-day world. Marie thoughtfully covers a wide breadth of topics important to clinicians and students of herbal medicine intent on becoming sex-positive stewards of the plant world. Not meant as a solution or quick fix for sexual or reproductive concerns, this book instead teaches how to weave the pleasures of plant medicine into daily life for both our healing and our happiness."

— DR. MARISA MARCIANO, ND, author of *The Botanical Medicine Manual* and chair of the botanical medicine department at the Canadian College of Naturopathic Medicine – Boucher Campus

The
Intimate
Herbal

A BEGINNER'S GUIDE
to Herbal Medicine *for* Sexual Health, Pleasure, *and* Hormonal Balance

MARIE WHITE

North Atlantic Books
Huichin, unceded Ohlone land
aka Berkeley, California

Published by
North Atlantic Books
Huichin, unceded Ohlone land
aka Berkeley, California

Cover art © gettyimages.com/saemilee;
gettyimages.com/Alex Livinsky
Cover design by Jess Morphew
Book design by Happenstance Type-O-Rama

Printed in the United States of America

The Intimate Herbal: A Beginner's Guide to Herbal Medicine for Sexual Health, Pleasure, and Hormonal Balance is sponsored and published by North Atlantic Books, an educational nonprofit based in the unceded Ohlone land Huichin (*aka* Berkeley, CA) that collaborates with partners to develop cross-cultural perspectives, nurture holistic views of art, science, the humanities, and healing, and seed personal and global transformation by publishing work on the relationship of body, spirit, and nature.

North Atlantic Books' publications are distributed to the US trade and internationally by Penguin Random House Publishers Services. For further information, visit our website at www.northatlanticbooks.com.

MEDICAL DISCLAIMER: The following information is intended for general information purposes only. Individuals should always see their health care provider before administering any suggestions made in this book. Any application of the material set forth in the following pages is at the reader's discretion and is their sole responsibility.

Library of Congress Cataloging-in-Publication Data

Names: White, Marie, 1991– author.
Title: The intimate herbal : a beginner's guide to herbal medicine for
    sexual health, pleasure, and hormonal balance / Marie White.
Description: Berkeley : North Atlantic Books, [2022] | Includes
    bibliographical references and index. | Summary: "A guide to making
    all-natural reproductive wellness remedies to enhance sexual health"—
    Provided by publisher.
Identifiers: LCCN 2021052806 (print) | LCCN 2021052807 (ebook) | ISBN
    9781623176631 (trade paperback) | ISBN 9781623176648 (ebook)
Subjects: LCSH: Herbs—Therapeutic use. | Reproductive health. | Sexual excitement.
Classification: LCC RM666.H33 W458 2022 (print) | LCC RM666.H33 (ebook) |
    DDC 615/.321—dc23/eng/20211202
LC record available at https://lccn.loc.gov/2021052806
LC ebook record available at https://lccn.loc.gov/2021052807

1 2 3 4 5 6 7 8 9 KPC 27 26 25 24 23 22

To calendula, damiana,
and the other plant guides
who walk with me

Contents

Introduction

Welcome to your complete holistic guide to supporting sexual and reproductive health with herbs, naturally. In *The Intimate Herbal,* you will dive deep into your capacity for sensuality, libido, fertility, and embodied pleasure through the help of healing herbs and herbal practices. *The Intimate Herbal* is also intended as a resource and guide for herbalists, naturopaths, nutritionists, therapists, community educators, and health advocates, along with complementary and alternative health therapists. As a health practitioner who wishes to guide your clients toward better sexual and reproductive health, you will find easy-to-follow and foolproof herbal and lifestyle wisdom in the following pages. This book will become a treasured addition to the herbal library with its strong focus on medicinal herbs to fold into your practice and add to your holistic tool kit.

This herbal was created as a pleasure-centered resource in which the promotion of sexual and reproductive wellness is given center stage. Daily preventative practices and habits that cultivate a healthy approach and relationship to sex and fertility are offered along with specific protocols that address health conditions with herbs. While other herbals published in the past have opted for a solution-oriented approach with a strong focus on undesirable health imbalances and illness and the right herbs to fix them, in *The Intimate Herbal* we get into the flow of a different health paradigm. Folks today don't have to wait to get sick or ill before they turn to herbs and bring healing herbal allies into their lives. Herbs work best when they are enjoyed regularly, supporting the body in gentle ways. Sensual and pleasurable health-enhancing herbal rituals are yours to adopt at any time. A health paradigm that no longer focuses on illness changes everything and opens up new ways of being healthy and well.

In the twenty-first century, offering an herb as a single remedy for a complex health problem like endometriosis or low sperm count can seem overly simplistic and out of touch. It can also perpetuate the belief that, rather than being multifaceted, health issues may be the simple result of a lack of herbs. It's undeniable today that chronic health conditions are on the rise. This is especially true in the realm of sexual and reproductive health, where the now common experiences of infertility, pelvic pain, and hormonal imbalances can no longer be considered individual abnormalities.

Growing up in the 1990s and coming into the herbal community in the early 2000s, I often felt there was something missing from my herbal training and herb books. Most of my teachers were older folks who had been trained by herbalists who came of age in a different era, a simpler time. Today, reasons why some people might experience sexual and reproductive challenges are not so simple or easy to pinpoint. An herbal methodology that focuses on the elimination of symptoms often comes at the expense of addressing their true root cause, some of which may be metabolic, systemic, or environmental. I've been working in herbal education for a decade now and have been in close contact with hundreds of students as well as leading herbalists that have shared my concerns and confirmed my suspicions. I've come to realize that we are ready for a different way, ready for an herbal practice that is more inclusive, more aware, and more grounded in the world we live in today. Working with medicinal herbs now ties into a wider commitment to health and wellness that brings together individual health, collective health, and the health of the planet. On this path, pleasure leads the way.

The guide you hold in your hands has been years in the making. It compiles over a decade of herbal study and practical, hands-on experience in the world of natural health, body literacy, somatics, sex and cycles, activism, ethnobotany, and medicinal herbs. My approach to herbalism, both as a teacher and as a practitioner, is to blend together folk traditions resting on centuries of traditional use along with the more modern lens of scientific discovery. The herbal protocols and plant monographs included in *The Intimate Herbal* rest on the folk herbalism recipes and traditions as they intersect with solid clinical evidence of safety and efficacy. In the spirit of curating a resourceful herbal focused on sexual and reproductive wellness,

I've included thorough herbal protocols for specific health conditions. These include herbs and protocols for such conditions as erectile dysfunction, irregular menstrual cycles, herpes, low libido, breast cysts, prostate cancer prevention, and much more.

While fertility and sex are covered at length from an herbalist's standpoint, the stages of pregnancy and birth are mostly skimmed over in this guide as they require a different set of herbal tonics and practices altogether. The materia medica included in these pages covers full-spectrum aphrodisiac herbs, sexual tonics, hormone balancers, liver cleansers, adaptogens, and other botanicals with a strong affinity for the sexual and reproductive organs and their associated systems for people of all genders. Finally, I've included relevant information around cultural uses of herbs and ecological considerations along with guidance on such concepts as regenerative agriculture, consent, intimacy and relationships, and lots of juicy sex-positive pleasure-as-liberation inspiration steeped in medicinal herbs and lore.

There are hundreds of herbs readily available to us today. The abundance of options can be daunting. In order to develop a simple, effective, and reliable framework for supporting sexual and reproductive wellness with herbal medicine, this book offers you a concise selection of healing herbs, seaweed, and fungi to choose from. These potent herbs and therapeutic substances will become your new sensual allies along this journey. Outside the realm of herbs, *The Intimate Herbal* also grows from a commitment to health and access to sexual and reproductive wellness as it relates to community advocacy. Herbalism doesn't exist in a vacuum, and as many of you work to reclaim health and healing through herbs, my hope is that the vitality you find as you go along will fuel your desire and ability to be involved in making sexual and reproductive health and herbal medicine accessible to those who need it.

My goal is to offer you a simple framework for working with herbs and for delving into herbal medicine. This book is accessible to anyone interested in sexual wellness and integrative health. No prior herbal background is necessary to read and learn from it. Accessibility, ease of use, and pleasure are core principles of the intimate herbalism practice laid out in these pages. I will guide you along herbal rituals, tips, tricks, and recipes that are so enjoyable and easy to follow that they're guaranteed to make compliance a breeze. These are healthful, pleasurable remedies people really want to be indulging in, over and over again. Apply them for yourself and your kindred others, your community and the folks you choose to nurture and care for, and for those who may come to you as clients to seek herbal guidance and advice.

The popularity of herbs and herbal remedies is booming across the globe, especially in developed countries where herbalism is trending. In light of this, I've gone against the grain and included a chapter on ways *not* to use herbs as medicine. Herbs, seaweed, and fungi are living organisms that are part of rich, active ecosystems. They need specific natural conditions in which to grow and thrive. Mixing and matching holistic strategies and nourishing tools like forest bathing, rest, and play along with herbs will transform your herbal lifestyle into a truly sustainable, regenerative practice.

Interactions with medication, contraindications, safety concerns, and personal preferences may also lead certain folks to seek herbal alternatives on their health journey. In the chapter "When Not to Use Herbs," you'll learn about nature connection, rest, sexological bodywork, community education, microdosing, and flower essences as they connect to sexual and reproductive health.

It's easy to see why interest into the world of healing herbs is booming today. In a fragmented world that celebrates busyness, the slow pace and seasonal realm of the natural world is healing in itself. The practice of using plants to keep the body in a place of harmony brings health and balance in more ways than just in a physical sense. Rather, when you work with medicinal herbs, you experience their healing touch on your body as well as your heart, spirit, and psyche.

Humans have a deep and ancient connection to the earth and the plants that inhabit it. Cultures around the world have been steeped in plant lore and traditional remedies that stem from every bioregional habitat and terroir. Even if you have never used herbs for healing or pleasure, your ancestors have. Reconnecting with herbs can be a way to honor your lineage and reconnect with your culture and its medicines. Plants, seaweed, and fungi have lived alongside us since time immemorial.

Folks starting on their herbal journey often experience something very real and embodied when they start working with herbs. This includes a sense of connection, of belonging, and intimacy with the world at large. When you welcome healing herbs and plant-based practices into your life, you develop empathy for your kindred others, a leaning toward nurturance, and a desire to be of service to the plants themselves, their natural habitats, your fellow humans, and yourself. This is the web of human and nonhuman connection that leading somatic sex educator Caffyn Jesse calls the "biosphere of belonging."[1] Herbs act as a gateway for unlocking pleasure and cultivating intimacy.

A journey of transformation unfolds when you blend the study and practice of herbalism together with a commitment to support sexual and reproductive wellness. All of us suffer in some way from the impact of sexism, inequality, medical bias, stigma, exposure to toxins and chemicals, and lack of sexual education and body literacy, starting at a young age and continuing all through life. But there are plant allies to discover that have an innate connection to the sexual and reproductive organs and their associated systems.

Sexual tonics and aphrodisiac herbs also benefit the nervous system, the hormonal system, and psychoemotional health. Herbs like tulsi, damiana, and milky oats inspire sexual vitality, stress regulation, hormonal balance, and mood lifting. These herbs and many more are covered in much detail throughout the following pages and can be enjoyed in endless varied forms, such as herbal infusions, baths, soaks, and nourishing drinks. The reclaiming of sexual and reproductive health, pleasure, and ease is not an ultimate destination but rather a lifelong pursuit. I look forward to walking that path with you, with *The Intimate Herbal* as our luscious road map.

Chapter Overview

Foundations of Intimate Herbalism

Clear overview of herbalism and its rich history, the difference between folk herbalism and the modern biomedical model of assessing herbal properties and actions, and a review of modern herb research and science.

When Not to Use Herbs

Sustainability of herbalism, activism, rest and play, sexological bodywork, community education, microdosing, flower essences, and the safety of herbs along with possible interactions.

Becoming an Intimate Herbalist

Herbal properties and benefits. Mastering the art of herbal preparations: extraction techniques and methodology, delivery systems, solvents, and ratios.

The Intimate Herbal Pharmacy

Herbal extraction methods and recipes: infusions, decoctions, drying, powders, syrups, herbal wines, herbal baths and soaks, oils and salves, liquid extracts, and herbal chocolates.

Sexual and Reproductive Health

Understanding sexual and reproductive health and function, including physiology and associated systems along with a short introduction to relevant herbs.

Intimate Health Conditions

Conditions relevant to intimate health and the sexual and reproductive organs, along with clear guidelines for herbal protocols complete with dosage, applications, modes of action, and delivery.

Intimate Herbal Materia Medica

A deep dive into intimate herbs and aphrodisiac, adaptogen, tonic, nervine, nutritive, and hormonal herbs that support sexual and reproductive health, and an in-depth exploration of selected healing herbs, seaweed, and fungi.

Intimate Herbal Recipes

And finally, a compendium of healing recipes using intimate tonics, from warm elixirs to syrups, breast oil, medicinal energy balls, bath blends and soaks, herbal infusions, and delicious therapeutic cacao-based treats.

I

Foundations of Intimate Herbalism

An Introduction to Herbalism

Herbalism is the art, science, and embodied practice of medicinal plant-based healing. Nutritious, therapeutic herbs support and enhance health, assist with symptom management, and in some cases reverse disease or infection. When symptoms of disharmony, illness, and imbalance occur, herbalists and herb folks reestablish balance and homeostasis, prevent complications, and lead the body back to harmony with the help of healing herbs and simple yet transformative herbal protocols.

Medicinal herb allies covered in this book include popular tonics like schisandra, shatavari, maca, red raspberry leaf, nettle, damiana, and oats, along with seaweed and algae as well as fungi such as cordyceps and reishi. These healing substances have been used around the world for hundreds (and in some cases, thousands) of years. More recently, modern science and clinical studies confirm their traditional uses in the realm of sexual and reproductive health. Herbalists become experts in plant-based alchemy, allying with medicinal herbs as guides and teachers. From this relationship steeped in respect and care comes the ability to match plants with people, and to find the right plant ally for someone at a given physiological, psychoemotional, and energetic level.

The practice of herbal medicine empowers folks to take a proactive and engaged approach to their health and well-being and that of their family and close ones. It's easy and rewarding to grow a garden big or small that offers nourishment and healing. You can make quick forays into trails and backyards that abound with wild therapeutic edibles; nettle, wild rose, and forest mushrooms all come to mind. And for those who don't seek or have the capacity to grow or harvest your own medicinal herbs, you can rely on suppliers and manufacturers of high-quality and high-integrity herbs and herbal extracts.

Home-based herbalism fills the kitchen and pantry with potent herbal remedies inspired by the seasons. As you become more intimate with the recipes and ingredients in the herbal kitchen, you will find comfort and ease with the herbal preparations that once seemed intimidating or confusing. Inspired herbal medicine-making integrates seamlessly into the weekly flow of your kitchen. Once you start making simple plant remedies at home, you will soon find yourself with a simmering pot of mineral-rich decoction lazily bubbling on the stove while you measure out seeds and berries to soak in a liquid extract for the next month. You will do these new tasks with the same familiarity with which you previously warmed a pot of soup for lunch or measured flour for muffins.

Homemade herbal medicines blend elegantly into the natural pantry and the daily flow of holistic meal preparation. I will share my favorite recipes and tips from the intimate herbal kitchen with you in the hope that your shelves will soon be stocked with the raw ingredients and vibrant medicines you need to become your own healer. As you'll learn throughout this book, supporting sexual and reproductive health with herbs can be simple and delicious.

Herbalism Today

Many people practice home herbalism as a hobby and lifestyle. Others pursue higher education in the field in order to gain a better understanding of herbal interactions, active compounds, and remedy formulation. In my experience working with numerous students of herbal medicine, I found that many folks are drawn to herbalism after a diagnosis of chronic illness or following a brush with conventional medicine. They look to herbalism for answers and seek empowerment through herbs. Integrative herbal medicine makes a perfect complement to conventional medicine. Increasing numbers of doctors are now training in herb and drug interactions to better counsel their patients in reducing medication dosage with the help of healing herbs. Health practitioners and clinicians trained in herbalism rely on clinically tested herbs for effective symptom management rather than symptom-suppressing drugs that may carry numerous risks and side effects.

Many new parents turn to herbalism when they raise their little ones. Herbs enable them to nurture and care for their babies and their growing families with healing natural remedies they can count on. Other folks are curious about herbalism after studies in botany or biology, led by their love and wonder for the natural world and its nonhuman inhabitants. Many people today desire to serve a purpose in their community by being herbalists. Community herbalists plant urban or rural healing gardens, craft small-batch herbal remedies, start grassroots botanical apothecaries, and provide one-on-one consultations with clients. Community-based herbalism incorporates healing foods and medicinal plants, kitchen-based medicine-making, and access to plant cultures. In this way, community-based herbalism fosters and nurtures relationships with self, others, places, and plants.

Plant medicine is people's medicine. Many folks are not able to rely on conventional medicine for treatment. Migrants and marginalized people may not have access to health coverage or health insurance. Others may not be comfortable visiting doctors' offices, such as stigmatized groups like indigenous people, LGBTQ+ people, racialized people, those with fat bodies and disabled bodies, or those with a history of medical trauma. The practice of herbalism is both empowering and a lifesaver. Medicinal herbs grace our days in the form of weedy walks, colorful herbal infusions, and healing powders sprinkled into warm drinks. They are steeped into flower-filled baths, sewn into dream pillows, and rubbed over the skin by loving hands.

History of Herbalism for Sexual and Reproductive Health

Humans have used plants for healing since time immemorial, passing down herbal knowledge from generation to generation via drawings, stories, folkloric tales, and songs. Medicinal herbs have been enjoyed for sexual and reproductive health throughout history and across countless cultures. The role of healer was often played by older women, the local crones who were responsible for the herbal harvest, remedy-making, midwifery, and tending to the sick. Throughout time, women harvested herbs and prepared healing potions. These day-to-day herbal practices were later compiled into written texts by men. That's why today, the history of herbal medicine (and botany, and gynecology, and medicine, among others) seems to be dominated by male voices.

Queer ecologist and plant scientist Sophie Duncan has explored the erasure of women's contribution to ecology and the study of herbs. She points out that the search for the terms "Father of Botany" brings up many notable names, while the search for "Mother of Botany" comes up blank.[1]

Our foremothers might be missing from standard literature, but we can nonetheless acknowledge their influence and thank them for keeping herbalism and plant healing alive for thousands of years. Archaeological excavations provide indirect evidence of early plant use. At the Saskatoon Mountain site in northwestern Alberta, Canada, in the wild boreal region, carbonized medicinal herb seeds were unearthed from a hearth alongside charcoal dated from more than nine thousand years ago. The carbonized seeds included species of raspberry, wild rose, and uva-ursi (bearberry) that are still used by herbalists in the context of sexual and reproductive health today.[2]

Written records about medicinal plants, on the other hand, date back at least five thousand years to the Sumerians, who described well-established therapeutic uses for plants like laurel, caraway, and thyme.[3] One of the oldest medical texts known today is the Kahun Papyrus, written by the Egyptians around 1800 BCE. A reference for early gynecology, it offers practices for fertility, pregnancy, childbirth, and contraception.[4] Descriptions of healing herbs still used today include cedar, elderberry, fennel, and peppermint.

Around 2700 BCE, Emperor Shen Nong was the second of China's mythical emperors and is widely considered the father of Chinese medicine. He cataloged over 365 species of medicinal plants and is believed to have personally tasted many of them. In the *Shen Nong Ben Cau Jing*, he writes of managing erectile dysfunction with ginseng root.[5] The word *ginseng* is derived from the Chinese term *rénshēn*, which translates to "man root." Ginseng is among Emperor Shen Nong's long-lasting contributions to herbal medicine. He recommended it for erectile dysfunction and to stimulate sexual appetite.

In Ayurveda, the ancient medicine that originated in India over three thousand years ago, a special class of *rasayana* tonics are known as *vrishya* to promote vitality and *vajikarana* to enhance libido. The concept of *vajikaran* as a libido tonic has been defined in the *Rigveda* and the *Yajurveda*, the first written texts of Ayurvedic medicine.[6] Vajikarana herbs are also the basis for therapies recommended in the *Kama Sutra*, the classic textbook for sex, intimacy, and pleasure between lovers and intimates. Vajikarana herbs include the adaptogens shatavari and ashwagandha.

In the fourth century BCE, the plant silphium, a sort of giant fennel and member of the carrot family (Apiaceae), is described as a potent and effective contraceptive.[7] It is believed that the Greeks and Egyptians used it as a contraceptive as early as the seventh century BCE on the advice of physicians. The plant was so widely used for food and medicine that it is rumored to have soon gone extinct, circa 300–400 BCE. Hippocrates (460–370 BCE) later described the use of wild carrot as another effective plant-based oral contraceptive.[8]

Hildegard von Bingen (1098–1179), a twelfth-century German abbess, is considered the first female doctor of the Catholic Church. She was a woman of great influence and power during her time and was held in high esteem among powerful religious and political figures. She wrote

extensively about women and particularly about gender differences, reproductive health, and sexual nature. Hildegard wrote about many herbs still
used today, such as hops, ginger, and licorice.[9]

Between 1450 and 1750, brutal witch trials unfolded in Europe. Between
75 and 85 percent of the accused were women. It is believed that many of
the women who were suspected of witchcraft were folk herbalists, healers,
and midwives. Some historians have disputed the claim that women healers were likely to be accused of witchcraft, pointing out that folks of various
backgrounds had been victims of the witch hunts. But nevertheless, the
thousands of women who died at the stake took with them to the grave a
wealth of folk healing and herbal knowledge, including herbs and herbal
practices related to sexual and reproductive health that may have been lost
forever. According to conservative estimates, 110,000 witch trials unfolded
in Europe during this dark and tragic period, out of which 40,000 to 60,000
resulted in executions.[10] Many scholars believe the number of unofficial
trials and their total death toll to be much higher.

Indigenous people occupying the land now known as North America
(Turtle Island) possess extensive knowledge of medicinal herbs for pregnancy, childbirth, and the postpartum period.[11] For example, common
yarrow *(Achillea millefolium)* is used by the Kwakiutl people of the Pacific
Northwest Coast as a poultice applied to the breasts after childbirth. The
roots of wild rose, on the other hand, are boiled and taken internally as
a decoction during the postpartum period, presumably for its astringent
and tonifying effect on the uterus. Blue cohosh and black cohosh are other
herbs commonly used in modern midwifery that date back to traditional
indigenous midwives for use during late pregnancy and labor.

Phytotherapy and the use of herbal remedies for health and healing
is returning to mainstream culture in North America today after a short
period of obscurity precipitated by the rise of allopathic medicine in the late
1800s and 1900s. During this time, much effort and money were invested
into discrediting herbal medicine as "old wives' tales" and "old wives' remedies" in a move that both bolstered patriarchy and sexism in medicine[12]
and also succeeded in shrouding herbalism under an air of quackery in the
collective mind for over a hundred years.[13] All of us herb folk celebrate the

renewed popularity of herbal medicine today with pints of nettle tea and celebratory armfuls of fireweed and mullein stalks. But as herbal medicine makes a resurgence, it's important to keep looking at the way the history of herbalism is skewed. Some herbalists continue to be ignored for their contributions. This includes indigenous herbalists, Black and brown herbalists, and queer and trans herbalists.

Herbal Studies and Research

As herbalism evolves well into the twenty-first century, new clinical studies and research complement the old traditional models of experience and observation. Before the microscope was invented, herb folk learned from the plants themselves. Herb-curious people watched animals and noted their use of herbal medicine. Herbal knowledge appeared in the form of dreams, visions, and hallucinations. People relied on stories, myths, traditions, and folk theories like the doctrine of signatures.

What Is the Doctrine of Signatures?

The doctrine of signatures offers a way to observe plants and make connections about their properties and uses based on their appearance, texture, feel, preferred habitats, and other sensory observations. Ethnobotanists have suggested that the doctrine of signatures may have been more of a technique for remembering plants and practicing the muscle of observation rather than a trusted technique to establish their medicinal value.

This may seem quite provincial and unscientific today, but modern science is now confirming a significant number of traditional herb uses that were gathered and passed down from hundreds and thousands of years of observation, experience, and inner intuition. Of course, as with any other discovery made throughout history, some of the early superstitions and beliefs around herbal medicine have later been proved to be wrong. But the use of visions and dreams to gain valid information and knowledge about the natural world was and continues to be a sound approach in many herbal traditions.

Maya healer Elijio Panti (1893–1996) exemplifies this traditional knowledge well.[14] His student Rosita Arvigo, a respected herbalist, ethnobotanist, and traditional healer, documented their mentoring journey in her 1994 book *Sastun: My Apprenticeship with a Maya Healer*. A Chicago native and rain forest transplant, she was lucky to be accepted by the respected healer and to learn under his tutelage despite her lack of Maya ancestry. Don Elijio was a student in the oral tradition that had been passed down from Maya healers for thousands of years. He could not write nor read, but possessed profound and intimate knowledge of the plants around him. In his eighties and nineties, he was instrumental in the ethnobotanical research focused on medicinal plants in Belize in a joint research project between the Belize Ethnobotany Project, the Ix Chel Tropical Research Foundation, the New York Botanical Garden, and the U.S. National Cancer Institute.[15]

Following her immersive education with Don Elijio, Arvigo would go on to create the Arvigo Method for Maya Abdominal Massage, incorporating healing elements from her training. This type of massage, now known as Arvigo Massage, is used for relieving a variety of sexual and reproductive complaints. Arvigo Massage may help effectively relieve chronic pelvic pain, menstrual irregularities, uterine fibroids, prostate swelling, erectile dysfunction, and infertility, along with helping break down adhesions and scar tissue from endometriosis.

Hortence Robinson (1923–2010) was another traditional healer and mentor to Rosita Arvigo.[16] Born on Cozumel island, the ancient home of the Maya goddess of medicine Ix Chel and where the Maya had their school for midwives, Hortence was a living library of knowledge about medicinal plants. She was a specialist in gynecology, obstetrics, and pediatrics; delivered thousands of babies; and also worked as a family physician. Hortence was invited to speak and teach in front of medical doctors, PhDs in public health, and nurse-midwives at the New York Academy of Medicine. Other engagements brought Hortence to the University of Massachusetts, Carnegie Mellon University, the National Cancer Institute, the Women's Herbal Conference, the International Herbal Conference, and the New

York Botanical Garden. Hortence gained much of her knowledge by observation and experience of the natural world. Dreams and visions taught her which herbs to use and how to prepare them.

While scientific advances have contributed widely to the field of herbalism by making herbal treatment more accessible to those who practice conventional medicine, much is lost when science dismisses the more intuitive aspects of herbal practice as primitive and esoteric. An approach to herbs that ignores the experience, tradition, and conceptual framework of traditional herbalism in favor of double-blind clinical trials and pharmacological studies alone is likely to yield conflicting results. This is happening currently with the emphasis on active ingredients and constituents along with isolated, standardized compounds from plants.

Extracts made from synthesized plant molecules are believed by some to be safer and more effective than traditional folk preparations made from the whole "crude" plant. A current prevailing view holds that herbal products can be therapeutic and safe only when the active ingredient is isolated, identified, standardized, and subjected to appropriate clinical studies, as if thousands of years of use didn't amount to an indication of safety and efficacy. But this belief and its subsequent trials led to the disappointing conclusion that herbs are often clinically unreliable. After all, any herbalist can tell you that an herb's qualitative and quantitative chemical composition varies with its region of origin, growing conditions, harvest time, method of processing, the part of the plant used (stems, flowers, leaves, buds, or shoots), and how long the harvested plant was stored before use.

Beyond chemical composition, each person responds differently to an herb and an herbal protocol based on their constitution, personality, and current acute or chronic conditions. That is part of what makes the science of herbalism so hard to capture via the framework of clinical data and metrics. It is also part of what makes herbalism a true art. I continue to be humbled and awed by the modern scientific research that validates what our elders and ancestors intuitively knew to be true.

The rich and intricate web of communication and chemistry that exists within the natural world connects plants and humans in magical and mysterious ways. Some relationships and interactions between plant cells and human cells have been proved while others have not. As this mystery unfolds, plants, seaweed, and fungi continue to act as healers and teachers. Whether or not you choose to work with plant remedies that have been proved or that remain unvalidated by science is a personal choice. Beyond ingesting medicinal herbs in therapeutic doses, other options for herbal therapy include nature connection, growing medicinal herb gardens for rest and enjoyment, and drop-dosing botanicals. These and more are covered in juicy detail in the next chapter.

2

When Not to Use Herbs

Integrated Herbalism

Herbalists have a vast tool kit at their disposal to amplify wellness and bolster positive change within the body without relying on therapeutic doses of medicinal herbs. Herbal medicine doesn't exist in a vacuum, and herbs have the deepest, widest impact when they are used synergistically with other rituals and tools. Integrated herbalism includes restorative practices like nature connection, sexological bodywork, and microdosing and drop-dosing. Think of these supportive additions as the active cultures that make the ferment come alive. Without them, herbs have to work that much harder to reach desired results, but together, they ignite and elevate their potency and benefit. If you suffer from burnout, exhaustion, and low libido, for example, you might benefit from a nervous system tonic like milky oats and a mineral-rich herb like nettle. However, before turning to herbs, you might implement a practice of afternoon naps, short daily walks, and cutting back on work hours if possible. You might acknowledge that we live in an era when overwork is worn like a badge of honor, and you might commit to reclaim, little by little, your right to rest and leisure. After all, sometimes people don't need herbs. Rather, sometimes what people really need is time off from work, connection with friends, a social media detox, a walk in nature, a mediator, a warm meal, a support group, affordable housing, a conversation.

In the context of sexual and reproductive health, the practice of integrated herbalism is especially valid. The best aphrodisiac herbs don't replace the hands of an attentive lover. A steaming cup of cacao elixir doesn't replace voice, consent, and desire. Sexual tonic herbs don't replace safe access to reproductive health care from educated and socially aware practitioners. Unprocessed trauma from rape, from miscarriage, or from a difficult abortion, and the rejection of family and friends based on sexual orientation, won't be healed by herbs alone. By focusing on herbs as medicinal and healing agents, we might forget and overlook the medicine that surrounds us always.

Everything is medicine. Herbs are medicine in the same way that nature is medicine, water is medicine, and air is medicine. Community is medicine, love is medicine, time is medicine, sex is medicine. Learning, art, rest, travel, kissing, crying, and long walks all carry the potential to be therapeutic in the same way herbs do. Herbs, flowers, seaweed, and fungi need not be your only teachers and allies.

Sustainability and the Earth

One of the many reasons why you may seek to reduce overreliance on botanical extracts as healing agents to offset sexual or reproductive imbalances has to do with the sustainability of herbs. Unlike other market products and consumer goods, herbs aren't made by machines in factories. Rather, they grow in natural habitats that are becoming scarcer by the minute. The voracious appetite of humans for medicinal herbs has driven many species to extinction, and many others stand on the brink. Numerous herbalists have a pantry full of herbs that they may never use and will eventually toss in the garbage. Beyond the individual level, herbal manufacturers also produce huge amounts of waste as part of the manufacturing process. But all of these factors become minuscule when compared with the loss of habitat worldwide due to climate change, resource extraction, and industrial development that threaten herbal communities. When using herbs to heal, we must view them as allies and companions rather than as our saviors.

One of the best approaches to creating stronger relationships with herbs is to grow them or forage them yourself. Even in the absence of land to call your own, community gardens may be available (and if not, why not start one?). My dad used to have a large yard brimming with garden herbs, fruit trees, nut trees, and grape vines. When he sold his house and downsized to a small apartment with no room to garden, he added his name to a neighborhood community garden waiting list. The sound of crickets ensued, so he resorted to guerrilla gardening. Along the train tracks near his new home, he scattered nettle seeds and planted rose bushes and heirloom apple trees. But it's not the reward of the harvest that he's after; rather, it's the medicine of growing plants.

Foraging is a good way to connect more deeply with the herbs as well. When it comes to foraging in the wild, be respectful and mindful. Keep a low footprint. It's best to keep your foraging to areas you know well, areas you return to year after year. This way, you can observe and measure your impact on the plant communities and ensure that your harvest is sustainable. Wild abundant weeds like nettle, cleavers, plantain, and dandelion are great foraging herbs because they are resilient and thrive in a variety of environments. As such, they are great companions to foragers. Sometimes the right foraging practice involves only admiring the plant without harvesting it. Time spent in nature is medicine in itself. Clinical herbalist Larken Bunce teaches that nature time reduces neuroendocrine hyperactivation, regulates allostatic mechanisms, and acts as a resourcing tool to help center oneself.[1]

Herbalism and using herbs to heal does not have to be unsustainable. Some herbs do grow in staggering abundance, and certain growing methods are inherently more sustainable than others. At the root of unsustainable herbalism is an attitude of entitlement, a belief that herbs exist to serve us, to heal us. But plants have agency of their own. They've been on this earth much longer than us humans. We have to unlearn this pattern and remember that we exist within a strong context of anthropocentrism that colors the way we interact with the world around us, including within the context of herbal medicine. Anthropocentrism is the belief that human beings are the most important entity in the universe, and it views other entities in relation to how they interact with or offer value to humans. Some folks find a valuable alternative and antidote to the dominant system in the form of deep ecology or ecocentrism, an ecological political philosophy that promotes a nature-centered system of values.

Nature-centered systems celebrate and recognize the inherent worth of all living beings, including plants, wild weeds, and medicinal herbs, regardless of their instrumental utility to human needs. Ecopsychology is another emerging field that honors and recognizes the role that nature plays in our health and well-being as a species. Beyond deep ecology and ecopsychology, the growing field of ecosexuality, or ecosex, promotes the exploration of the places where ecology and sexology intersect (hence the cool term *sexecology*). A term coined by ecofeminist scholars Beth Stephens and Annie Sprinkle, sexecology shifts our relationship to the earth away from "earth as mother" and more toward "earth as lover."[2] The concept of earth as lover invites you to swim naked in rivers, to spend time with nature, to appreciate and caress and protect it, and not to take it for granted. It reminds us that connecting with the natural world is inherently sensual.

Herbal activism becomes a part of rewiring our connection to herbs, of shifting our perspective. Some folks grow native flower gardens just for the bees. Others grow wild medicinals for wildlife: for deer, butterflies, bears, and birds. Some grow bioremediating mushrooms to help cleanse and revitalize the ground. Folks grow elaborate gardens as meditative spaces. Gardens can be just a place for people to go and relax, and not to harvest anything from. Capitalism has us believe that anything that doesn't earn a buck is worthless. This mentality is leading us to spiritual, cultural, and environmental collapse.

As more people become aware of the many ways we can interact with herbs in a therapeutic way that doesn't involve buying and consuming them, we open up a whole new way of engaging with herbalism and with the world around us. We all have the innate ability to connect deeply with plants and with the earth. More than any infusion, extract, or herbal consultation, this relationship may be the real medicine at work. Herbal medicine is sensual and embodied and cultivates intimacy both within and without.

Rest and Play

When I was growing up, my family and I spent a few summers backpacking around the world together. We traveled by bus and boarded ferries to faraway places where few travelers had ever set foot. This was a time before cell phones, before widespread internet, and many of the small villages we stayed in lived in the traditional ways they had been accustomed to for hundreds of years. I was shocked and delighted to realize that, from the mountains to the desert, through the ancient and quiet ocean-side towns, and across the continents, folks living in traditional ways all shared one thing in common: they loved to rest and play, and they did it often.

They sat in the sun or in the shade; they invented games to pass the time, played dice, played ball, and chitchatted for hours with neighbors across the fence. I had been taught in school that ancestral ways and primitive ways of living relied on endless chores and tasks necessary for survival that left no time for rest and leisure, but here was proof that just the opposite was true. People in those villages liked to sit and enjoy the weather and each other. Kids, adults, and elders alike sat on benches and watched the animals ambling along, the insects crawling near, and they listened to the wind blow. Since then, I've held on to the value of rest and play as essential human needs that enable us to grow intimate with the world around us, with one another, and with ourselves.

Holistic protocols for sexual and reproductive health include rest and play alongside herbs and, in some cases, in the place of herbs. Rest triggers a cascade of stress-reducing hormones, a slower heart rate, enhanced digestion, deeper breathing; it relaxes stiff and tense muscles and promotes the release of natural painkilling endorphins. Rest accomplishes this via activation of the parasympathetic nervous system, which down-regulates the sympathetic nervous system and shifts the body away from fight-or-flight and into rest-and-digest. Switching off the activity of the sympathetic nervous system enhances sexual function. Nocturnal erections are a good example of this. Nocturnal erections occur primarily during rapid eye movement (REM) sleep, the stage associated with dreaming. Women also experience episodes of nocturnal arousal when the sympathetic nervous system is at rest.[3] During REM sleep, women experience the ebb and flow of labial, vaginal, and clitoral engorgement. Play, on the other hand, relieves stress and improves brain function, boosts creativity, and builds stronger connections and relationships to others.

The impact of rest and play as a core practice for sexual and reproductive health is well demonstrated by how relaxed and aroused you can feel while on vacation, away from the daily responsibilities and stresses associated with the busy schedules many of us have come to accept as normal. If time constraints are an issue, or if the idea of resting or playing for any amount of time during the day feels like something you can't make space for, you can start small and go from there. Ten minutes a day of rest or play is an amazing place to start and builds a solid foundation over time. For those with more spacious schedules, consider a bare minimum of an hour a day, one day a week, and one week a year as time dedicated to rest and play.

Some of my own commitments to rest include daily afternoon naps, for which I've set up a few different soft and cozy day beds and nap spots around my house, along with a commitment to daily neighborhood walks. From a religious and spiritual perspective, Buddhism, Judaism, Christianity, and Islam all practice a holy day of the week devoted to prayer, rest, and the absence of work and technology. My family and I used to rest every Sunday after church, when the only pursuit worth doing that day was preparation of a delicious Sunday dinner, often cooked outside on an open fire—even on frigid snowy winter nights. The Sunday rest has fallen out of style lately, but our need for rest hasn't. Rest can take the form of naps, yoga, neighborhood walks, meditation, gardening, baking, or other activities that bring your body and mind to a calm, relaxed, and happy place.

Play can be anything from dancing, card games, kitchen experiments, and playful group activities to crafts, along with anything else that can be done for fun rather than for profit or gain. Educational games are all right, but don't dismiss plain old play for the sake of play with no further agenda either. It helps if you have allies and comrades in this, like partners, kids, friends, parents, pets, neighbors, and other folks interested in the pursuit of rest and play as life practices.

My own commitments to play include a bake-off every Monday, when our ten or so neighbors gather for our weekly "family dinner." Each week I challenge myself to bake some over-the-top dessert for the occasion, and add new recipes to my repertoire as a play practice that brings me joy and pleasure—not to mention that it brings pleasure to the dinner guests and their palates as well. Some recent highlights include an inverted maple flan and a three-layer lemon meringue pie on an almond flour and date sugar crust. Next, I want to tackle homemade baklava with a homemade flaky crust, honeyed pistachios, and rose water.

Another of my commitments to play as a life practice is the yearly tradition that my partner and I share of going to the Okanagan Valley in British Columbia, Canada, on a wine tour every summer. We visit vineyards all afternoon, eat delicious picnics on our favorite nude beach, and fall in love all over again with ourselves, with each other, and with life. It's just a few hours from home, but it feels as luxurious as a villa in Tuscany. Sustainable embodied herbalism includes the medicine of rest and laughter. Practice it with a full heart, and practice it often.

Sexological Bodywork

Sexological bodywork, also called somatic sex education, is trauma-informed body-based sex therapy. Educators trained in somatic sex education offer experiments and experiences to bring alive and nurture the sensual self. They use tools like breath, movement, sound, and touch. Areas of focus in the realm of somatic sex education include enjoyment, consent, the anatomy of pleasure, sexual expression, and sexual identity. Unlike conventional sex therapy and talk therapy, somatic sex education can include one-way sexual anatomy touching, sexual pleasure, and orgasm. Somatic sex coaches teach that conscious erotic touch can bring about states of consciousness and wisdom that can only be accessed through pleasure and through the lens of clear sexual energy.

For those who need more than talk therapy or medicinal herbs alone, somatic sex education unwinds sexual wounds in the nervous system, releasing patterns of trauma and neglect through embodied practices like breath, movement, sound, and healing sexual touch and pleasure. You can find somatic sex educators or sexological bodyworkers along with more information and training opportunities in this field of study at the Institute of Somatic Sexology in Australia as well as at the Institute for the Study of Somatic Sex Education, based in Canada.

There are many opportunities to blend together herbal medicine and somatic sex education in the healing of health challenges like erectile dysfunction, lack of orgasm, pelvic pain, postpartum recovery, premature ejaculation, and sexual trauma. Along with body-centered mindfulness, breathing exercises, and attentive touch, medicinal herbs and sexological bodywork relax the body, soften the heart, and bring blood flow to the genitals for healing and pleasure.

Community Education

Community education and body literacy play an important role in sexual and reproductive health. Experiences of fertility, sex, and cycles can transform not just bodies but entire lives. Honoring both science and spirit, many folks are ready to claim their pleasure and power in their sexual bodies and to help others do the same. Folks drawn to the work of intimate herbalism include herbalists, doulas, midwives, acupuncturists, bodyworkers, sexologists and somatic sex educators, counselors, nurses, yoga teachers, fertility awareness instructors, and health practitioners as a whole.

Becoming educated on sexual and reproductive health includes exploring topics like contraception and conception, anatomy, womb care, hormonal health, prevention and treatment of sexually transmitted infections (STIs), sexuality and pleasure, communication, consent, boundaries and desires, and full-spectrum prenatal, childbirth, postpartum, miscarriage, and abortion options and care. Community educators teach workshops and classes, print zines and booklets, offer mentorship and learning programs, join podcasts, write blogs, organize get-togethers, and share their passion and knowledge through many media.

My own budding interest in herbal medicine was nurtured when, at the age of seventeen, I was gifted a small zine with a bright pink cover called

Hot Pants: Do-It-Yourself Gynecology and Herbal Remedies. The zine was offered to me by my roommate Pam, a student in creative arts therapies at Concordia University in Montreal. The worn cover and soft dog-eared pages suggested the zine had been well used, passed from hand to hand among a circle of women who surrounded me and would become my long-wished-for mentors. This grassroots booklet, one of many of its genre, was compiled by Isabelle Gauthier and Lisa Vinebaum. I own the forty-eight-page 1999 edition produced by the Blood Sisters, but there are many other editions in circulation.

My copy has traveled back and forth across the country many times and, with Pam's scribblings and notes on the back cover, is still a valued resource in my herbal library. Sure, after more than a decade of advanced herbal studies and practice, I find many of the basic recommendations in the booklet to be somewhat rudimentary and incomplete. But the effect this zine had on me at a time when all of this information was new, inspiring, and revolutionary is one that is enduring and continues to guide me today.

Organizers and educators who offer their guidance in a trauma-informed, resilience-based, nonjudgmental, inclusive, supportive, and empathetic way help counter the lack of sex education and conversation around sexual wellness. Options abound for sharing and partaking in the gospel of sex and fertility education and sovereignty. Opportunities for learning and for engaging with kindred others is part of reclaiming sexual and reproductive health. Community education plays an essential and often inspiring and pleasurable role in this process.

Microdosing and Drop-Dosing

The concept of a right dosage for medicinal herbs is elusive. This is part of the reason why large-scale clinical studies on the effects of medicinal herbs can have conflicting results, whereas the individual protocols found in traditional use in which dosage varies tend to have more consistent results. The right dosage for medicinal herbs depends on the individual, on the herb used, on the season, on the mood, and many other tiny, complex, and rich factors that have more to do with intuition and inner knowing than with theory.

Where larger medicinal herb doses bring a physiological impact to the body, drop-doses rather bring an emotional and energetic quality to their action. Larger doses will take you there, but drop-doses are like an invitation to the party. Medicinal herbs with an affinity for drop-dosing include nervines and aphrodisiacs. Passionflower, damiana, reishi, and rose are some of my favorites to drop-dose and can be enjoyed as single drops of tincture or liquid extract placed on the tongue. The sensual experience of drop-dosing with an herb can be more potent than a larger dose diluted in a glass of water. The taste and presence of the herb is somehow multiplied as the dose is reduced. Handcrafted small-batch herbal remedies often carry more potency in that regard when compared with store-bought remedies that tend to be produced with less vibrant plant material.

Microdosing and drop-dosing medicinal herbs may appear to be similar to using flower essences, but the two practices are different. Flower essences are diluted in water many times over, resulting in an energetically potent remedy that looks and tastes like water. Drop-doses of herbal liquid extracts, however, maintain their full sensual qualities. Colors brighten, aromas weave through the air, texture fills your mouth, and taste dances on your tongue.

The concept of microdosing also applies to healing substances like psilocybin mushrooms, fungi, cacti, and other mind-altering and mood-shifting botanicals, which are currently being investigated for sexual health and healing. Experiences with sacred plant medicines can be a tool to increase sexual pleasure and relationship satisfaction. Some researchers are investigating MDMA for the healing of sexual trauma, psilocybin for the treatment of sexual dysfunctions that are psychological in nature, and ayahuasca as an aid to bring together sexuality and spirituality. Medicinal herbs with psychoactive potential in the realm of sexual healing also include cannabis and blue lotus.

Cannabis and CBD formulas can enhance arousal, sexual intimacy, and pleasure. Endocannabinoid receptors are present throughout the nervous system and the endocrine system, and in the sexual and reproductive organs. On a microscopic level, endocannabinoid receptors are connected with nerves that relay sensations, immune cells that tweak inflammation, glands that govern hormone secretion, and muscles that encourage energy usage. Cannabis and especially CBD can treat painful sex and increase orgasms.[4] Dosage is important. A small dose can be stimulating, while high doses may be too sedating or intoxicating to promote good sex. For local application, vaginal and anal CBD suppositories are optimal.

Blue lotus contains the alkaloids aporphine and apomorphine, which show effects on dopamine receptors within the limbic system, the part of the brain largely associated with emotions and the emotional realm. Blue lotus has a long history of use as an aphrodisiac and has traditionally been enjoyed to increase libido, sexual appetite, and arousal. Nuciferine, another alkaloid in blue lotus, relaxes the nervous system, while apomorphine reverses the effects of erectile dysfunction by increasing blood flow to the penis. The ability of blue lotus to tone and relax the nervous system and to decrease stress and anxiety levels allows for easier and more profound orgasms.

Cannabis, blue lotus, and other mood-altering aphrodisiacs don't need to be specifically used for sex. Enjoy these herbs and their rituals as a gateway for building a sensual relationship with yourself, with spiritual forces, and with creativity. These herbs and substances invite increased sexual awareness into your life. Sexual energy generates and propels inspiration, rejuvenation, passion, self-love, creation, and Eros as life force.

Flower Essences

Flower essences are vibrational remedies that act on the emotional and energetic body. Using the essence of fresh flowers, and at times other healing substances like seaweed and mushrooms, flower essences recalibrate thought patterns and support healing pathways beyond the physiological effects of herbal extracts. Flower essences make a great companion to traditional herbal remedies as an adjuvant to bolster the effects of a formula. At times, flower essences are the first remedy of choice. Many herbalists and herbal practitioners blend together herbal extracts in their traditional form with the addition of essences.

When dealing with health and wellness, and patterns of imbalance and disease, the body is connected to the mind, the emotions, the soul, the inner longings, people and places, and so many other factors that are invisible to the eye. The concept of mind-body connection, once relegated to the "alternative" realm by mainstream medicine, can no longer be ignored as a fabrication. In scientific terms, the mind-body connection is referred to as the biopsychosocial model, which is both a philosophy of care and a practical guide to health and wellness.[5] Lifestyle, stress, health beliefs, and social conditions like cultural influences, family relationships, and social support have an impact on the body and its physical functions. Communication networks connect the brain and the neurological, endocrine, and immune systems.[6] Nowhere is this intimate web of connectedness more apparent than in the realm of sex, fertility, and cycles.

Under stress—be it environmental stress from pollution, physical stress from poor nutrition, emotional stress from loneliness or grief, or mental stress from overwork and systemic inequality—the brain initiates a cascade of reactions involving the hypothalamic-pituitary-adrenal (HPA) axis, which is the primary actor of the endocrine stress response. This increases the production of steroid hormones called glucocorticoids, which include the stress hormone cortisol. Excess amounts of cortisol disrupt the normal biochemical functioning of the sexual and reproductive system.

Chronic stress affects testosterone production, decreases sex drive and libido, causes erectile dysfunction and impotence, and lowers sperm quality. High levels of stress also disrupt the menstrual cycle, increase the likelihood of painful menstrual cramping and premenstrual syndrome (PMS), extinguish sexual desire, worsen menopausal symptoms, and even flare up preexisting conditions like herpes and polycystic ovary syndrome (PCOS).[7] Flower essences show up as valuable allies when navigating the stresses associated with sexual and reproductive disorders such as dysmenorrhea, endometriosis, prostate cancer, and infertility.

Sex, love, intimacy, and desire are loaded with emotions. Gender dysphoria, experiences of chronic sexual issues, and trauma from abortion, stillbirth, or miscarriage linger in the sexual and reproductive organs as well as in the psyche. This causes disruptions and imbalances that physical remedies, which act primarily on a physiological level, cannot access, cannot work with, and cannot heal. But flower essences and vibrational remedies are uniquely suited to the emotional and energetic aspect of these experiences, helping to reestablish balance. For best results, match flower essences with other healing modalities like therapy, support groups, and integrative health care.

Flower essences are made from fresh and vibrant plant material that soaks and extracts for a few hours in water placed next to the mother plant, usually on a sunny summer day or under the light of the moon. The essence is then strained, removing the plant parts and particles, and is mixed with alcohol for preservation at a ratio of 1 to 1. This mother essence is then diluted through a process of dilution and activation. Herbal essence practitioners vary in their dilution ratios, with some folks using the mother essence as a remedy while others dilute the essence upward of seven times, concentrating its effect and potency away from its physiological action and more toward its energetic action.

Flower essences tap into the healing nature of plants, fungi, and other natural substances. They are healing and therapeutic in a similar way that a stroll in a beautiful flower garden and a walk in the woods is healing to the heart and psyche. Different plants and flowers carry different signatures, which then interact with our own human signature and work to soothe, inspire, protect, and uplift.

Though popular essences coming from Europe have come to be regarded as the most prevalent in flower essence therapies, there is a lot of value in engaging with local flowers, plants, seaweed, and fungi. Based on where you live, local small-scale makers of essences are using elements from your bioregion and ecosystem from which to make medicines uniquely suited to work with you.

One of the advantages of flower essences as an alternative or complement to traditional herbal medicine is that flower essences are safe to use at any time due to their dilution. Because they contain no active compounds in a physical way, flower essences may also be used in conjunction with medications such as anxiolytics, antipsychotics, and antidepressants as well as during pregnancy and breast-feeding, before and after surgery, and throughout chemotherapy treatment. In this way, flower essences are unparalleled as emotional allies that support sexual and reproductive health in myriad ways.

Safety and Interactions

When considering whether or not to use an herb or herbal protocol for health and healing, safety concerns and possible herb-drug interactions often come up as questions. In fact, herbs are generally safe when taken in their recommended dosage and as advised by experienced and knowledgeable herbalists. The incidence of interactions between herbal medicines and nutritional supplements with conventional drugs is low.[8] Currently there is no reliable information available to draw upon when assessing the scale of any possible problem or harm, or for predicting solid clinical outcomes. Even in the case of St. John's wort, which is now commonly known to interact with a number of drugs, including the contraceptive pill, the clinical significance of some reported cases cannot be accurately evaluated due to the variation in the nature of the herb itself and products made from it.

An interaction reported from a concentrated and standardized plant extract does not necessarily apply to the same whole crude plant in smaller doses. The lack of evidence when it comes to negative interactions between herbs and medications may be due to underreporting or unrecognized interactions. But there is also the possibility that many herbal medicines have a generally safe profile and do not interact significantly with drugs. Interactions may occur between prescription drugs, over-the-counter drugs, dietary supplements, and even food. Many positive interactions have been identified, and other negligible interactions have been noted. Negative interactions of clinical significance are rare.

Aside from a few well-known examples, concerns about herb-drug interactions are often not based on rigorous research. Most herb-drug interactions identified in current sources may be hypothetical, inferred from animal studies, cellular assays, or based on other indirect means. Well-designed clinical studies evaluating herbal supplement–drug interactions are limited and sometimes inconclusive.[9] It is also noticeable that, while anecdotal or theoretical evidence is quite rightly considered unacceptable as evidence when it comes to proving the efficacy of herbal products, the same anecdotal and theoretical evidence seems to be given undue credibility when arguing the potential toxicity of herbs. Consumers as well as practitioners of natural medicines have observed this double standard.

However, it also doesn't mean that all herbs are safe all the time. While some herbs are gentle and nourishing in nature, other herbs are potent substances that have strong effects on the body. When it comes to herb-drug interactions, the main concerns come down to two possible pathways of interactions: pharmacokinetic interactions, or pharmacodynamic interactions.

Pharmacokinetic interactions consist of an herb possibly affecting the processes by which drugs are absorbed, distributed, metabolized, and excreted (the so-called ADME interactions). An important mode of action for this reaction is the liver's CYP-450 enzyme system, as numerous medications, nutrients, and herbal remedies are metabolized through it. This system can be either inhibited or induced by drugs or herbs. Once altered, there can be clinically significant interactions that may cause unanticipated adverse reactions or therapeutic failures.

Pharmacodynamic interactions, on the other hand, are those where the effects of one drug are changed by the presence of another drug (or herb) at its site of action. Sometimes the two might directly compete for particular receptors, but more often the reaction is more indirect and involves interference with physiological mechanisms. They include such reactions as additive or synergistic reactions, also called potentiation, where substances with similar effects are added together, or antagonistic or opposing reactions, where the substances cancel each other out. For example, two substances with sedative effect may potentiate and make the user extra sleepy. Alternatively, one substance may be stimulating while the other is relaxing. The two substances may cancel each other out, leaving the user neither stimulated nor relaxed.

Those who are most at risk of herb-drug interactions include the elderly, due to potential reduced liver and renal function, as well as folks who take drugs with a narrow therapeutic window such as anticoagulants and immunosuppressants. During pregnancy, only gentle and pregnancy-safe herbs should be used, and most commonly in the form of food. When combining medications and medicinal herbs, talk to your doctor, naturopathic doctor, pharmacist, or psychiatrist about your use of herbal remedies. But be aware that the majority of health providers do not know herbs well and are not trained in herb-drug interactions.[10] Surveys have shown that 75 percent of doctors queried admitted they had little to no knowledge about herbs. Meanwhile, 81 percent of pharmacists from an international cohort felt they had inadequate skills or knowledge to counsel patients on herbal remedies. As a result of their limited knowledge or lack thereof, they may counsel patients to avoid medicinal herbs altogether.

Other doctors and pharmacists uneducated in herbalism go even farther and claim that herbs are either worthless or very dangerous. Though they may be well-trained and educated in their respective fields of expertise, they know little about herbs and are ill equipped to make such statements on the subject of herbal medicine. As such, their statements should not be taken too seriously. Even extensive naturopathic studies include only a short introduction to phytotherapy. This makes naturopathic doctors under-resourced for herbal recommendations as well. The same goes for psychiatrists, as the benefits of herbs and possible interactions between medicinal herbs and psychiatric drugs are not covered in psychiatry coursework. In conclusion, I recommend that folks who use both prescription medication and herbal remedies work with a collaborative team consisting of a clinical herbalist to complement the support of their health practitioners. This will allow for a well-rounded, informed, and effective care team for matters of sexual and reproductive health.

3

Becoming an
Intimate Herbalist

Why Make Herbal Preparations

Making simple and delicious herbal preparations at home is easy and rewarding. Tapping into the therapeutic powers of aphrodisiac herbs, adaptogens, nervines, and calming herbal allies can be as quick as whipping up a batch of tea or folding some herb powders into drinks. Food and medicine blends into one in the herbal kitchen, and pleasure and flavor take center stage. I know of no better medicine than the handcrafted remedies I can imagine and bring to life in my herbal kitchen and the healing and enjoyment they bring to me and my friends.

Making herbal preparations from scratch by yourself may seem hard and intimidating at first. The first few batches of remedies you make may turn out to be disappointing. But all you need is a bit of practice. Time and dedication are an essential part of learning the herbal medicine–making process. Medicine-making is a lost art. Many advanced herbal students as well as herbal practitioners possess extensive intellectual knowledge of plants while having very little embodied hands-on experience of turning plants into medicine from scratch. When it is done right, kitchen-based herbal medicine offers unparalleled remedy quality, freshness, and potency.

However, a few rules and tips must be followed in order to make quality herbal preparations. All of these and more are found in the following pages. In this chapter, you will learn about herbal terminology along with the primary herbal actions relevant within an intimate herbal practice that centers on sexual and reproductive health, fertility, and cycles. This is essential herbal knowledge you will equip yourself with before you confidently work with herbs and herbal extracts and start building your own intimate herbal pharmacy.

Herbal Terminology

A basic understanding of herbal terminology, systems, and tools is essential in order to work with herbs in a therapeutic way. At the core of common herbal terminology are herbal actions and properties. Herbs have a wide range of actions on the body. A single herb can have numerous actions, while some herbal actions may work synergistically. In this section, brief descriptions are offered for important herbal concepts, including herbal categories, actions, properties, and constituents.

Herb Categories

Herb categories include such groups as culinary herbs, medicinal herbs, safe herbs, low-dose herbs, toxic herbs, at-risk herbs, local herbs, exotic herbs, and more. Herb categories are vast and varied, and many herbs from separate categories may overlap.

Culinary herbs are aromatic herbs with a strong history of use as flavoring agents and in cooking. Culinary herbs taste good and are potent medicinals. Some of them are also low-dose herbs. Examples of culinary herbs include rosemary and fennel.

Medicinal herbs may not be suited to culinary use due to their strong tastes and are prepared in concentrated extracts instead. Medicinal herbs are rich in active constituents such as alkaloids, terpenoids, saponins, phenolic compounds, flavonoids, and tannins, which influence their actions, properties, and tastes. Examples of medicinal herbs include calendula and goldenseal.

Safe herbs can be taken in large amounts and over long periods in relative safety and without negatively impacting organ function. They possess no negative interaction with food or medications and can be enjoyed by children and elders as well as during breast-feeding. Examples of safe herbs include nettle and milky oats.

Low-dose herbs are meant to be taken in small therapeutic doses. In larger doses, they may pose a risk to certain organs or alter mood and consciousness. Examples of low-dose herbs include cacao and vitex.

Toxic herbs range from mildly toxic to potentially deadly. They may be medicinal in small doses and administered by herbal therapists, such as in the form of flower essences. Examples of toxic herbs include datura and poison hemlock.

At-risk herbs are exposed to a risk of extinction, often due to overharvesting or loss of habitat. Many medicinal herbs are considered at-risk in the wild, so it is recommended only to use them in their cultivated form or avoid them altogether by replacing them with more abundant herbal alternatives. Examples of at-risk herbs include wild American ginseng and wild cordyceps mushroom.

Local herbs are native to or well established in your environment. What constitutes local versus exotic depends on where you live. Choosing local herbs in your herbal practice can have many advantages, like having more control over or knowledge of how the herbs were grown and harvested (organic, fair trade) as well as supporting the local economy.

Exotic herbs stem from foreign herbal traditions and grow in different climates across the globe. The healing herb and spice trade is an ancient and common practice, but it carries challenges when it is not done in an ethical way. At my home in British Columbia, Canada, I've recently started cultivating herbs that I previously considered to be exotic: schisandra and ashwagandha, which hail from Traditional Chinese Medicine (TCM) and Ayurveda, respectively.

Herbal Actions

Herbal actions are often used along with herbal properties. Action is the "what," and property is the "how." Herbal actions mentioned in this book are directly or indirectly related to sexual and reproductive health. Some of their common definitions:

Abortifacient herbs may induce miscarriage, especially in the first two months of pregnancy. They may be oxytocic or toxic.

Adaptogen herbs heighten resistance to stress and have an overall tonic effect.

Adjuvant herbs are used in conjunction with other herbs to increase their effect or to enhance a formula.

Alterative herbs are also known as depurative herbs. They are supportive remedies that gradually restore the body to a state of health and vitality.

Antidepressant herbs relieve depression. They may be a nervine, tonic, or adaptogen.

Antifungal herbs inhibit the growth of yeast and fungus.

Anti-inflammatory herbs relieve inflammation. They may be astringent or emollient.

Antioxidant herbs prevent and reverse free radical formation and oxidative stress.

Antispasmodic herbs are also known as spasmolytic herbs. They reduce cramping and spasms. They may be nervine or carminative.

Anxiolytic herbs soothe anxiety and reduce the intensity, severity, and frequency of panic attacks.

Aphrodisiac herbs enhance sexual desire and stamina. They may be tonic, adaptogen, or stimulant.

Aromatic herbs are often synonymous with carminative herbs. They are rich in aromas and contain essential oils responsible for a stimulating or relaxing effect.

Astringent herbs tighten tissues with a binding action on the mucous membranes. They reduce inflammation and irritation. They are often rich in tannins.

Bitter herbs enhance the digestive process and support liver health and pancreatic function.

Carminative herbs are rich in aromatic volatile oils that support digestion.

Cholagogue herbs stimulate the flow of bile from the liver. They may be bitter or hepatic.

Demulcent herbs are used internally. They are rich in mucilage, which soothes and protects inflamed internal tissue. When used externally, this action is known as emollient.

Depurative herbs are also known as alterative herbs.

Diuretic herbs increase output of urine and the excretion of waste through the kidneys.

Emmenagogue herbs stimulate and regulate menstrual flow. They may bring on a late period and should be avoided in early pregnancy.

Emollient herbs are used externally. When used internally or ingested, they are known as demulcent. They may contain mucilage or natural oils that soothe and protect the skin, tissues, and mucous membranes.

Hepatic herbs support liver health and help increase the flow of bile. They may be bitter or cholagogue.

Hormonal herbs are also known as hormone balancers. They contain plant constituents that affect hormonal function in the body and alter circulating levels of estrogen, progesterone, testosterone, luteinizing hormone (LH), follicle-stimulating hormone (FSH), and cortisol.

Hypnotic herbs are potent calming herbs and sedative herbs that induce deep sleep and rest.

Nervine herbs support the health and function of the nervous system. They may be tonic, stimulant, or calming.

Nutritive herbs are deeply nourishing and rich in bioavailable vitamins, minerals, amino acids, and other nutrients essential for good health.

Sedative herbs calm the nervous system; soothe stress, tension, and anxiety; and induce sleep when taken in larger doses.

Spasmolytic herbs are also known as antispasmodics. They reduce cramping and spasms. They may be nervine or carminative.

Stimulant herbs may be system-specific (for example, specific to the circulatory system or to the nervous system). They kickstart physiological activity in the body, whether as a circulatory stimulant, a nervine stimulant, an immune stimulant, or other.

Tonic herbs strengthen the body as a whole or a specific organ or body system (such as a nervous system tonic, a sexual tonic, or other).

Trophorestorative herbs are superior tonics with a strong affinity with a specific organ system, such as liver trophorestoratives or uterine trophorestorative. They restore optimal organ function.

Herbal Properties

Herbal properties are also known as modes of action. Properties of medicinal herbs expand on their physiological impact on the body, which leads to an herbal action. For example, an action of milky oats (*Avena sativa*) is to act as a nervous system tonic and soothe stress.[1] The herb's action is easy to notice and remember. The herbal property, on the other hand, digs a bit deeper into the "why." In this example, the herbal property of milky oats, or why milky oats act as a nervine, is associated with its MAO-B inhibitory activity, which is linked to the unique bioactive compounds avenanthramides.[2] These compounds play a role in the breakdown of neurotransmitters or chemical messengers like dopamine in the brain. The indole alkaloid gramine is also thought to be responsible for the gentle sedative effect of *Avena sativa*. In short, the herbal properties of herbs are tied to certain active constituents. The properties inform the action.

Herbal Constituents

Plants produce a wide diversity of secondary metabolites that serve as defense compounds and signal compounds.[3] In general, secondary metabolites exhibit a wide range of biological and pharmacological properties. In herbal medicine, these secondary metabolites are known as herbal constituents. Emphasis on single constituents as a way to explore how herbs deliver their properties is a relatively new development in herbalism and is centered within the practice of pharmacology.

Many traditional herbalists maintain that whole plant extracts are more potent than isolated active constituents. Each whole plant extract may contain dozens or even hundreds of constituents, often from several structural groups. In most cases, it is almost impossible to define a single constituent to explain the bioactivity of the herbal extract or its traditional application in herbal medicine. The activity of an herbal extract is due to synergistic interactions of several constituents present, which means that the effect of a plant extract cannot be determined by the evaluation of single compounds alone.

Therapeutic constituents in healing herbs include phenolic compounds (flavonoids, phenylpropanoids, rosmarinic acid, catechins, tannins, polyketides), terpenoids (mono- and sesquiterpenes, iridoids, saponins), and polysaccharides, among others. Each of these constituents possesses a wide range of actions, from antioxidant to anti-inflammatory to mood-enhancing activity. In other words, herbal constituents do not control single physiological effects but rather influence various receptors, pathways, feedback loops, and other biological reactions.

Sensual Observation

Herbs may taste sour, bitter, sweet, salty, pungent, and spicy. Sensual observation consists of noticing the texture of the plant and its scent, color, and other notable sensory characteristics. These observations help create a thorough plant profile to guide intuition and experimentation with herbs in a therapeutic way. In terms of plant constituents, plant coloring hints at the presence of certain phytochemicals. For example, yellow, red, and purple may signal the presence of flavonoids.[4]

Types of Extracts and Remedies

Liquid extracts are herbal extracts made from liquid substances. They are added to water, juice, kombucha, and food preparation; squirted on the tongue; drop-dosed; or administered in other creative ways of delivery. Liquid extracts are made in such solvents as water, alcohol, glycerin, vinegar, honey, mead, juice, or ferments. They offer color, taste, scent, and a truly sensory experience of connection with the herbs.

Food-based remedies are made with culinary and nutritious herbs. Food-based remedies include herbal powders stirred into homemade granola, sprinkled over lattes, or folded into salad dressing. Fresh spring greens and edible flowers are blended into pesto. Herbal vinegars are added to recipes, and herbal glycerites to drinks. The possibilities are endless. Food-based remedies demand an intimate understanding of herb tastes and blends.

Travel kits are important for those who have a busy lifestyle. Some herbal extracts and remedies are more travel-friendly than others. Capsules are the absolute best in terms of convenience for those who travel lots or are always on the move. Liquid extracts and herbal oils can leak and spill. An herbal travel kit is essential if you want to keep up with your herbal regimen while being away from home. Capsules hinder the sensual experience of herbal medicine, and as such they are at times shunned by the cognoscenti and herbal purists as an inferior method of delivery. But even the best tincture in the world is no use to you when you're squeezing it out of your clothes after it's spilled all over your luggage on the plane.

Chronic condition remedies are meant to be taken continually and over long periods. Chronic health conditions (the opposite of acute conditions) require a steady supply of gentle herbs in formulas that are enjoyable and fit well within your lifestyle. Because they are meant to be used daily over many weeks and months, making them pleasurable is a top priority.

Acute condition remedies are herbal extracts meant for short-term use. Acute formulas are often fast-acting and potent. In this way, they differ from remedies made to address and work with chronic deep-seated conditions. Remedies meant for acute conditions taste strong and work fast. Liquid formulas work best for this, especially for pain. They start working as soon as they touch the tongue. Many herbs used for acute conditions are rich in secondary constituents and should not be taken long-term.

Curative remedies are made with a specific intention in mind: enhancing organ function, reducing inflammation, or other action that serves to support health and healing on a physiological level. Unlike pleasure remedies that can be taken just for fun, curative remedies serve a clear purpose and are not always pleasant to consume. Curative extracts may be formulated via the folk method or the clinical method. But not all the remedies in your intimate herbal pharmacy have to be curative (see "Pleasure remedies," below).

Pleasure remedies earn a place of choice in your intimate herbal pharmacy. Make them or use them because they taste and feel great. I like to offer "tincture tastings" when friends and loved ones come to visit my home: we go through the whole collection drop by drop. I explain what this herb and that will do in the body. Inevitably, when we get to the pleasure remedies, people ask, What's this one for? I reply, "That one is just for fun." People love them, and it reminds them that pleasure is medicine.

Etheric extracts (drop-doses) exist on a different continuum from physiologically curative remedies. In essence, etheric extracts offer the experience of tiny, homeopathic doses of herbal extracts or remedies that tap into emotional and energetic patterns rather than the physical body.

Clinical extracts are the curative extracts as validated by science as active and therapeutic. Clinical extracts are made according to exact measurements and ratios so that active constituents are clearly quantified by dosage. Made via the clinical method rather than the folk method, clinical extracts are often made by manufacturers or herbal clinicians for use in herbal therapy.

Art of Extraction and Delivery

From the time humans started using herbs to heal, they have devised ways to keep medicinal herbs fresh for longer. The quest for the most reliable, potent, and long-lasting herbal preparations likely began with water extractions, which are done at air temperature and with few tools.[5] Water is a universal solvent and extracts many soluble constituents from plant material.

Other ancient and accessible preservation techniques include wild ferments made with medicinal herbs. Local wild flora has been used as a fermented beverage starter culture for thousands of years across the world. Where water infusion and handcrafted ferments sit at one end of the extraction spectrum as simple and low-tech techniques, many more elaborate extraction methods have been devised by modern medicine-making manufacturers in order to get the most medicine out of each plant.

Herbal extraction process types range from simple maceration, infusion, decoction, and percolation to more elaborate Soxhlet extraction, microwave-assisted extraction, and ultrasound extraction. For home herbalism, simple extraction methods are sufficient and reliable. For larger companies and organizations, high-tech extraction allows a potentially more economical and ecologically friendly approach to medicine-making, as less plant material is needed per final product.

The advantages of home-based herbal extraction include accessibility of equipment (standard kitchen tools will work), the ability to work with a large variety and high quality of herbs and solvents like organic plant oils and local honeys, and the liberty to craft remedies in small batches. Folk herbalism is the medicine of the people, and reclaiming the art of medicine-making and herbal extraction is a step toward health and community sovereignty, not to mention it is also creative and fun. The practice of home herbalism helps decentralize knowledge and wellness from the hands of a few large herbal companies and back into the hands of local herbalists, farmers, and community folk.

Some of the challenges associated with large-scale herbal manufacturers are that although some of them do produce large quantities of high-quality and high-integrity herbal remedies, many others may be governed by profits rather than by a commitment to the local economy, ecological restoration, the potency and vibrancy of the herbs and remedies, and the health of those who consume them. That being said, large-scale herbal manufacturers and the high-tech extraction techniques associated with a bigger and more controlled production model offer many advantages too, especially for herbal clinicians and practitioners of collaborative medicine bridging together conventional allopathic and alternative holistic treatments.

The scientific method of herbal extraction is required for all commercially sold herbal extracts. The scientific method requires more time and equipment, but it allows for better-quality testing, more consistent extraction, and standardization, and it can be reproduced exactly from one batch to the next.[6] These are important considerations in a therapeutic context, as herbal extracts made with the scientific method can more adequately be assessed for potency and safety.

Whether it is done on a small or large scale, the art of herbal extraction and delivery rests on a few techniques and tools and includes a choice of solvent, extraction process, formula, and intake.

The solvent, also called menstruum, is the substance in which the plant will be extracted and preserved. Common solvents in folk herbalism are water, alcohol, oil, honey, and vinegar. The choice of solvent depends on the type of plant, which plant part will be extracted, the nature of the bioactive compounds in the plant, and the intended use of the final herbal extract.

The process of extraction is most often via hot or cold infusion or maceration, which can take anywhere from just a few hours to a full month or moon cycle. The extraction itself is mostly a hands-off process once the tools and material have been thoroughly washed and sanitized and the right plant part and solvent have been combined.

Once the extraction is complete, the herbal formula comes into play along with the final product and its desired intake. Will the decoction be turned into a syrup? The oil into a salve? Or maybe single tinctures will be blended into a custom formula. In the following section, you will find more information about solvents, ratios, herbal formulas, and types of extracts, along with instructions and recipes for the main herbal preparations used within the context of intimate herbalism for sexual and reproductive health.

Solvents and Ratios

The plant parts used within the context of herbal extraction include fresh or dried plants: roots, leaves, flowers, seeds, pollen, plant oils, or resins and gums. Nutritional components of plants include sugars, amino acids, proteins, fats, vitamins, macrominerals and trace minerals, and chlorophyll. And finally, secondary metabolites (also called secondary plant constituents) for herbal extraction include alkaloids, terpenoids, saponins, phenolic compounds, flavonoids, and tannins, among others.

Common Solvents

WATER

Water is a common solvent for herbal extraction. Advantages of using water as a solvent are that it is readily accessible and low-cost compared to other solvents like alcohol, and that water extracts constituents well. Known as a universal solvent, water is used in the extraction of a wide range of constituents, such as minerals, water-soluble vitamins (C and the B-complex vitamins such as vitamins B_6, B_{12}, niacin, riboflavin, and folate), and chlorophyll as well as polysaccharides, starches, and mucilage. As a solvent, water is accessible and nontoxic.

Some of the disadvantages of using water as a solvent for herbal extraction include the short shelf life of water-based herbal extracts. Water extraction does not preserve herbs for very long as it may promote bacterial and mold growth. Other solvents are required to help preserve the shelf life of water extractions. Another disadvantage of water as a solvent is that a large amount of heat may be required to concentrate the extract, as in the case of hot infusion or decoction. Water alone does not adequately extract essential oils and resins.

In terms of ratios for water-based herbal extraction, increase the ratio of herb to water when working with fresh herbs as compared to dried ones. Fresh herbs contain more water than dried herbs and are therefore less concentrated.

ALCOHOL

Alcohol is the best solvent for extracting secondary plant constituents. It has a wide range of extraction and it is an excellent preservative and sanitizer. Aside from extraction ability, other advantages of alcohol as a solvent include a long shelf life. Herbal extracts made in alcohol have a very long shelf life, which makes alcohol extraction more ecological and low-waste than other extraction methods.

The disadvantages of alcohol have to do with concerns like safety and cost. There are safety issues with alcohol-based herbal extracts, namely use with people who struggle with alcohol addiction or abuse, alcohol-sensitive folks, people who avoid alcohol for religious or cultural reasons, and those with liver disease or other medication interactions. You may also wish to avoid alcohol when administering herbal remedies to toddlers and children, during pregnancy and breast-feeding, and for elders. What's more, most commercially available alcohol is made from GMO corn, sugarcane, or sugar beets, so you may want to avoid it or source organic alcohol instead. There may be a strong alcohol taste to alcohol extracts, which some find off-putting. Finally, alcohol is expensive and less accessible in large quantities compared with water and lower-cost ingredients like vegetable glycerin and apple cider vinegar.

In terms of ratios for medicine-making, the minimum alcohol content needed to preserve herbal extracts and lengthen shelf life is a 1-to-4 or 1-to-5 ratio of alcohol to other solvents, or a percentage of 20–25 percent alcohol. Plants rich in resins and aromatic oils require a higher alcohol concentration for extraction.

VEGETABLE GLYCERIN

Food-grade vegetable glycerin is sourced from palm, soy, or coconut oil. A colorless, odorless, viscous fluid with a very sweet taste and low glycemic index, glycerin sits between water and alcohol in terms of solvent ability. Luckily, glycerin pairs well with both water and alcohol solvents for herbal extraction. Glycerin makes an ideal solvent for toddlers and children as well as those with an alcohol sensitivity or who avoid alcohol for personal, medical, or religious reasons.

Some of the previously mentioned advantages of using glycerin as a solvent may turn into disadvantages, however. Take the sweet taste, for example. The sweet taste of glycerin may be cloying when remedies are taken in high doses. When consumed in excess, glycerin can also dry out the throat, resulting in a sore throat. The dosage of glycerin-based extracts (called glycerites) must be higher than with alcohol-based extracts in order to compensate for the reduced extraction ability of glycerin. Finally, glycerites have a lower shelf life than alcohol-based herbal extracts.

For medicine-making, glycerin has about 50 percent of the solvent power of alcohol. When glycerin is blended with water, a ratio of 60 percent glycerin to 40 percent water is needed for preservation. A good ratio of glycerin to water for an herbal glycerite made from dried herbs is ¾ glycerin to ¼ water. When working with fresh and juicy herbs, 100 percent glycerin may be used. When extracting tannins in alcohol and glycerin, glycerin will hold tannins from precipitation. Along with helping to hold the herbal constituents in suspension in the formula, glycerin added to herbal tinctures enhances the taste by adding sweetness and mellowing the harshness of alcohol. When juicing fresh herbs, a 1-to-1 ratio, 50 percent glycerin to 50 percent fresh plant juice, will help preserve the juice.

APPLE CIDER VINEGAR

Apple cider vinegar is used to promote digestion and support liver health. Vinegar is about 4 percent acetic acid, which extracts some fat-soluble constituents. Vinegar as a solvent will also extract minerals well. Like glycerin, vinegar offers a useful alcohol-free alternative to those who wish to avoid alcohol.

The downside of using vinegar as a base for herbal extraction is that, like glycerin, it does not keep as long as an alcohol-based tincture and has a shelf life of three to six months. Vinegar does not extract as many constituents as alcohol either. The sour taste of vinegar may be off-putting to some. Finally, medicinal vinegars are best kept in glass jars with plastic lids, rather than the classic metal screw-on lid many home herbalists use, because vinegar will rust the lids over time.

Oxymels, an herbal potion that blends vinegar and honey, are a superb way to enjoy herbal vinegars and taste delicious. For oxymels, the ratio of vinegar to honey may be 1-to-2 or 1-to-1.

OIL

Olive oil, sunflower oil, hemp oil, or jojoba oil are good solvents for resins, oleoresins, essential oils, and flavonoids. Oil does not evaporate and is lighter than water. Oil-based herbal extractions mix well with resins and waxes for preservation. Herbal oils are typically made for external use, which means they are used on the skin as an oil or turned into salves with the addition of beeswax.

Oil can be a finicky solvent. Oil extracts are prone to spoilage on exposure to heat, air, moisture, light, and bacteria. Spoiled herbal oils have a rancid smell and taste. Oil does not mix with water or alcohol. In the making of a good herbal oil, make sure your plant material is completely covered with oil to avoid spoilage during the extraction process. Dried plant material is preferred for oil extraction, except for herbs that have to be used fresh.

Ratios of herb to oil for herbal extraction range between 1-to-2 (1 part herb with 2 parts oil) and 1-to-5, depending on the herb and whether it is fresh or dried.

4

The Intimate Herbal Pharmacy

Building the Intimate Herbal Pharmacy

In the following pages, you'll find guidance and instructions on how to make simple home remedies that have the potential to transform your sexual and reproductive wellness. With herbs as a blank canvas, it's possible to create a wealth of herbal remedies from a few simple ingredients. A well-stocked herbal pharmacy at home is an essential component of your herbal practice. Rather than finding, making, or buying appropriate herbal remedies when the need arises, it's best to always have a few key remedies on hand and at the ready. Like a kitchen pantry filled with your own favorite staples and essentials from which to assemble countless meals, the herbal pharmacy is different for every home and specifically designed to meet your own needs and preferences and those of your friends and family.

My herbal pharmacy has evolved over the years along with my learnings as an herbalist. These days, I favor tinctures and herbal baths as my go-to methods for herbal healing. As a result, my personal apothecary is laden with liquid extracts and whole dried herbs for soaks and baths.

I also grow and forage more herbs than in the beginning of my herbal immersion, as I've grown more comfortable with organic gardening and plant identification in the wild. My herbal pharmacy contains mostly homegrown herbs or locally foraged ones, with a few exceptions. I make a large variety of tinctures and extracts every year for my own use and to gift, trade, or sell.

Building your own herbal pharmacy begins with selecting the ingredients and extraction methods that best meet your needs and desires. The intimate herbal pharmacy will contain all your primary herbs and remedies for supporting sexual and reproductive health. Pick herbs in the materia medica that have the highest affinity with you and find them in dried herb form, as a liquid extract, in capsules, and other preparations for preventative and curative use. Sift through the following instructions on how to make classic herbal preparations and choose the ones that appeal the most to you.

Beyond tinctures and capsules, there are countless creative herbal remedies to be made and created at home. Syrups, powders, herbal chocolates, ferments, and elixirs all have the potential to be both yummy and therapeutic. When building your herbal pharmacy, essential components include whole dried herbs, herb powders, solvents and carriers like alcohol, glycerin, and honey, along with oils and healthy fats like olive oil and cacao butter.

Infusions, decoctions, powders, syrups, herbal wines, liqueurs, live ferments, baths, soaks, oils, salves, liquid extracts, and delicious herbal chocolates make up the intimate herbal recipe collection. Find inspiration and guidance on how to make herbal preparations and how to properly store herbs and remedies to maintain potency and freshness.

About sourcing herbs: many folks don't have access to wild places for ethical foraging, and many more may not have gardens in which to grow herbs. Others still may not have the desire, capacity, or inclination to craft their own herbal products. In light of this, you will also find recommendations on how to source herbs and herbal products from suppliers as well as key factors to look for in order to be an ethical and aware consumer of herbal medicine. Lastly, this chapter covers some herbal troubleshooting that goes over common reasons why herbs and herbal protocols at times don't deliver their desired results, and what to do instead.

Intimate Herbs and Full-Spectrum Aphrodisiacs

The herbs in the intimate herbal pharmacy are full-spectrum aphrodisiacs. Aphrodisiac herbs are defined as substances that stimulate sexual arousal, desire, pleasure, and performance. They work via a range of mechanisms affecting the brain, blood flow, and hormones. The word *aphrodisiac* is derived from Aphrodite, the ancient Greek goddess of love. Aphrodisiac herbs include pleasure herbs like damiana, cacao, maca, and shatavari. They typically possess aphrodisiac qualities and actions that apply to all genders, although specific herbs have a history of use with a specific gender, like shatavari associated with women in the Ayurvedic tradition, for instance.

Beyond classic aphrodisiac herbs, full-spectrum aphrodisiacs also include nervine herbs, adaptogen herbs, tonic herbs, nutritive herbs, and hormonal herbs. Potent, seductive herbs and herbal rituals are invited into wellness protocols, blending together soothing nervines and potent nutritive tonics along with seductive aphrodisiacs for a full-spectrum action on the body, mind, heart, and psyche.

The herbs in the aphrodisiac spectrum may not bring a direct action on the sexual or reproductive organs but rather bring a harmonizing quality to the body as a whole. They enhance the effect of aphrodisiacs and support sexual and reproductive health via an array of channels. In this way, nutritive tonics like nettle, aromatic digestives like ginger, and soothing nervines like milky oats become core herbs in a sensual herbal practice and a sensual life. Hepatics like schisandra and adaptogens like ashwagandha act as full-spectrum aphrodisiacs via their action on hormone regulation and heightened vitality.

Aphrodisiac Spectrum

Aphrodisiac herbs show up on a spectrum. Full-spectrum aphrodisiac herbs include nervine herbs, adaptogen herbs, tonic herbs, nutritive herbs, and hormonal herbs. These groups of herbs and their respective actions and properties are detailed in the following sections.

NERVINE HERBS

Nervine herbs have an effect on the central nervous system. Types of nervine herbs include nervine tonics or trophorestoratives, nervine relaxants, and nervine stimulants.

Nervine tonics (also called nervous system trophorestoratives) are potent stress and anxiety relievers. They strengthen and nourish the nervous system, and directly restore tissue health to nerve cells. Some adaptogen herbs are also nervine tonics, such as ashwagandha and reishi mushroom. Important nervous system trophorestoratives used in the context of sexual and reproductive health include milky oats and damiana.

Nervine relaxants, on the other hand, help relax and let go of tension in both a mental, emotional, and physical sense. They can be both nervine relaxants and antispasmodics, which soothe muscular tension. These healing herbs are great companions to aphrodisiacs, especially for the highly stressed, anxious, or tense individual. Nervine relaxants like passionflower help relax the busy mind, open the heart, and soften into a warm embrace. In high doses, however, many of these dose-dependent herbs can act as sedatives or hypnotics, so watch how much you take!

Nervine stimulants include cacao and other pleasure plants. Nervine stimulants directly enliven the sympathetic nervous system and act as circulatory stimulants, accelerate heart rate, increase blood flow, and boost short-term stamina and focus.

ADAPTOGEN HERBS

Adaptogen herbs support homeostasis, normalize body functions, and heighten resistance to stress. This action includes better resilience toward physical stress, emotional or mental stress, and even stress from environmental toxins and pollution. In other words, adaptogens reduce the impact of stress in a broad, multichannel, and nonspecific way. They won't overly tax specific organs or bodily systems. Rather, adaptogens support the body and mind as a whole. In essence, adaptogens are stress response modifiers. Adaptogenic herbs and fungi affect the hypothalamic-pituitary-adrenal (HPA) axis along with the immune-neuro-endocrine system.

Adaptogens like eleuthero, schisandra, and ashwagandha regulate cortisol production, strengthen the functioning of body systems, and enhance cellular energy transfer. This in turn helps the body utilize oxygen, glucose, lipids, and proteins more efficiently. In this way, adaptogens work completely differently than calming herbs like passionflower or nervine stimulants like cacao.

However, like nervines, adaptogen herbs also exist on a spectrum. Some adaptogens act to calm, build, and nourish while others work to stimulate and arouse. More calming adaptogens include ashwagandha, reishi mushroom, and holy basil (tulsi), while more stimulating and arousing adaptogens include eleuthero, ginseng, schisandra, and maca. Avoid stimulating adaptogens during exhaustion, burnout, and other states of depletion, for which trophorestorative nervines are more indicated.

TONIC HERBS

Tonic herbs have a broad action to strengthen an organ system or bodily system, and in some cases to strengthen the body as a whole. While tonic herbs are not necessarily nutritive, they do increase assimilation of nutrients. Tonics are often known as specific tonics, which means they are associated with a specific organ or bodily system.

Nervous system tonics include milky oats and damiana. Adrenal tonics include eleuthero, rhodiola, and ashwagandha. Lymphatic tonics include calendula, red clovers, and cleavers. Uterine tonics include red raspberry leaf, ginger, and vitex. Liver tonics include milk thistle, turmeric, schisandra, and reishi. Heart tonics include hawthorn and cacao. Sexual tonics include maca, ginseng, and cordyceps.

Aside from these examples of specific tonics, there are a few herbs known as general tonics. They impart a tonic action on the body as a whole. These are revered herbs and are often taken daily as part of an ongoing health and wellness routine. General tonics include reishi and nettle.

NUTRITIVE HERBS

Nutritive herbs (also called nutritive tonics) are herbs that offer a wealth of highly assimilable nutrients. They make the perfect addition to any health regimen and are often the first herbs recommended by herbalists to bring the body back to balance. They are often enjoyed in the form of herbal tea or infusions. They taste delicious and are safe to consume, even in high amounts.

Nutritive herbs include nettle, milky oats, and red raspberry leaf. Their generous vitamin and mineral composition makes them superb aphrodisiacs. Sexual and reproductive health, the sexual and reproductive organs, and the flow of hormones and neurotransmitters involved in sexual intimacy all depend on a steady stream of bioavailable nutrients supplied by nutritive herbs.

HORMONAL HERBS

Hormonal herbs can act as hormone balancers or hormone regulators. They balance and normalize endocrine function. While it's important to note that these herbs don't contain hormones, they rather act as hormone precursors or support the body toward better hormone regulation. In this way, some herbs can increase hormonal activity and influence reproductive hormones that in turn influence sexual desire and libido.

Hormones affect sexual and reproductive function in varied ways. Individuals with higher levels of testosterone experience higher levels of sexual desire, while estrogen levels affect vaginal lubrication. Progesterone, on the other hand, acts as an anaphrodisiac, lowering libido and sexual desire. Finally, the bonding hormone oxytocin intensifies orgasms and makes one feel more connected to their lovers or intimates.

Hormone imbalances, such as estrogen dominance, may increase the risk of thyroid dysfunction and infertility. Along with hormonal herbs, liver-supporting herbs (also called hepatic herbs) often have a regulating effect on hormonal activity. Hepatic herbs with an indirect action on hormonal health include milk thistle, dong quai, schisandra, and turmeric. Hormonal herbs include shatavari, damiana, saw palmetto, wild yam, vitex, and nettle root.

Full-spectrum aphrodisiac herbs include the following.

Ashwagandha *(Withania somnifera)* is a calming adaptogen beneficial as a long-term tonic. It provides relief from exhaustion and insomnia in support of a healthy libido and calm state of mind. Ashwagandha root has been studied for its fertility-enhancing effect, specifically as it relates to sperm quality.

Cacao *(Theobroma cacao)* acts as a stimulating nervine, increasing blood flow, stamina, and focus. Antioxidant-rich and cardioprotective, cacao delivers many compounds known to alter mood, lift depression and anxiety, and stoke romance. A potent therapeutic carrier in low doses, cacao and chocolate are the perfect vessels for medicinal herbs.

Calendula *(Calendula officinalis)* soothes inflammation and acts as a potent lymphatic tonic. A prime herb for inflamed mucosa, calendula oil or salve makes a perfect ally for the tender, sensitive tissues of the sexual organs. Taken internally, calendula acts as a depurative or alterative, assisting in the elimination of metabolic waste and enhancing lymphatic flow.

Cleavers *(Galium aparine)* is a gentle depurative and lymphatic with a strong affinity for the genitourinary system and the kidneys. A cleansing spring green, cleavers makes a potent anticancer extract, specifically for breast cancer prevention. It pairs well with calendula and red clover.

Damiana *(Turnera diffusa)* brings benefits to the nervous system as a nervine tonic that balances relaxation and excitement. The leaves of the aromatic shrub act as an antidepressant and anxiolytic to relieve depression and anxiety. Damiana is a celebrated aphrodisiac that soothes nerves and enhances mood in support of a healthy libido.

Dandelion *(Taraxacum officinale)* leaves and roots have potent cleansing activity along with supporting enhanced digestion and liver health. The leaves are nutritive and diuretic while the roots have strong hepatoprotective effects. Dandelion affects sexual and reproductive health indirectly via its action on body metabolism and general health.

Eleuthero *(Eleutherococcus senticosus)* is an adaptogen herb to increase stamina, energy, concentration, and focus. Also called Siberian ginseng, it improves resistance to stress and relieves the impact of physical stress, emotional or mental stress, and environmental stress.

Fennel *(Foeniculum vulgare)* is a soothing digestive and carminative that enhances the digestive process. Highly aromatic, fennel seed soothes spasms and cramping by acting as a spasmolytic. During breast-feeding, fennel increases milk flow and relieves colic.

Ginger *(Zingiber officinale)* is a warming aromatic spice and medicinal herb with an affinity for enhancing blood flow and circulation and relieving cramping. A prime ally for menstrual cramps and pain, ginger also soothes morning sickness during pregnancy. A circulatory stimulant, ginger awakens the senses and works as a tasty and therapeutic adjuvant in herbal formulas.

Ginseng *(Panax ginseng)* is a trusted adaptogen and aphrodisiac. Highly energizing and rejuvenating, ginseng is a potent ally with a strong affinity for elders and folks in their elder years. Ginseng supports healthy, strong erections and sexual intimacy. Avoid during burnout or exhaustion in favor of more calming adaptogens like ashwagandha or reishi.

Hawthorn *(Crataegus* spp.) is a prime heart tonic and cardiovascular system supporting herb. It pairs well with cacao and ashwagandha for promoting heart health both on a physiological and energetic level. It has a strong amphoteric and balancing effect on heart function and blood circulation.

Maca *(Lepidium meyenii)* provides highly bioavailable nutrition as a nutritive root enjoyed in powder form. Aphrodisiac and adaptogen, maca increases energy levels and helps maintain healthy libido and strength. It has been studied for its beneficial effect on fertility. Maca root enhances sexual function during menopause.

Milky oats *(Avena sativa)* provide intense nutrition in the form of vitamins and minerals like calcium, potassium, and vitamin C. Combined with hawthorn, milky oats work as a heart tonic and promote cardiovascular health along with healthy blood flow. An antidepressant and nervine tonic, milky oats are a superior ally for sexual and reproductive health.

Nettle *(Urtica dioica)* is a potent nutritive rich in calcium, magnesium, iron, and other minerals. It is a general builder and tonic that reverses fatigue, chronic conditions, and low libido. Nettle leaf is a nutritive tonic beneficial for whole-body health while nettle root has a strong affinity with the prostate and genitourinary system. Nettle seeds are trophorestorative to the kidneys.

Passionflower *(Passiflora incarnata)* is a relaxing nervine that soothes the nervous system and calms anxiety, repetitive and circular depressive thoughts, and pain in the body. Anxiolytic and antidepressant, passionflower benefits those who are too tired, strung out, anxious, and overworked to be their full sensual selves. It acts as hypotensive heart medicine to lower high blood pressure.

Red clover *(Trifolium pratense)* is a nutritive herb that is lymphatic, depurative, and a source of phytoestrogens. It is rich in isoflavones, flavonoids, phenolic acids, minerals, and saponins. Red clover is beneficial during menopause with its protective effects on osteoporosis and the cardiovascular system.[1] It is used for breast cancer prevention.

Red raspberry leaf *(Rubus idaeus)* tones and strengthens the uterus as a uterine tonic. A nutritive herb, it supplies essential vitamins and minerals for the optimal functioning of the sexual and reproductive organs. It pairs well with nettle leaf and ginger for uterine conditions.

Rose *(Rosa spp.)* is a beloved bloom long revered as a sensual plant. Antioxidant-rich and sweet-tasting, rose is a good heart remedy that awakens the senses and brings delight to the nose and tongue. It is astringent, with strong affinity with the skin and integumentary system.

Rosemary *(Rosmarinus officinalis)* is a stimulating herb acting on many channels. As a circulatory stimulant, rosemary supports blood flow and pairs well with *Ginkgo biloba* for erectile dysfunction. It is antioxidant, carminative, and bitter. Rosemary supports cognitive function and can act as a stimulating nervine.

Saw palmetto *(Serenoa repens)* benefits prostate health as a diuretic and anti-inflammatory to relieve acute and chronic prostatitis and benign prostate hyperplasia (BPH) or enlarged prostate when paired with nettle root extract. Saw palmetto also acts as a uterine tonic beneficial for toning the reproductive organs.

Schisandra *(Schisandra chinensis)* is an adaptogen and liver trophorestorative from Traditional Chinese Medicine that balances hormones via its action on hepatic function. Schisandra is an aphrodisiac and increases the quality, intensity, and duration of orgasms.

Shatavari *(Asparagus racemosus)* is an adaptogen and reproductive tonic with a strong affinity for the uterus and ovaries. Shatavari increases vaginal lubrication and is especially beneficial during menopause when estrogen levels decline. It is a nourishing tonic and aphrodisiac.

Slippery elm *(Ulmus rubra)* provides intense nutrition as a nutritive tonic and demulcent. Safe and rejuvenating, slippery elm can be taken safely by toddlers and other children, during pregnancy and breast-feeding, and by elders. Slippery elm is indicated during periods of convalescence, during postpartum, and to reverse depletion from exhaustion or burnout.

Tulsi *(Ocimum tenuiflorum)* regulates the stress response as an adaptogen. Also called holy basil, it's a prime remedy for those whose digestion suffers as a result of stress. The combined effect of stress reduction and enhanced digestive function makes tulsi a superb aphrodisiac and sexual and reproductive tonic.

Vitex *(Vitex agnus-castus)* harmonizes menstrual function and acts as a reproductive tonic. Also called chasteberry, vitex increases fertility in some cases and regulates the hormone cycle associated with pituitary function.

Wild yam *(Dioscorea villosa)* is a potent anti-inflammatory to relieve cramping and pain. Wild yam is a source of diosgenin, a potential building block for steroidal hormones such as progesterone. Spasmolytic and nervine, wild yam is commonly used for supporting reproductive function.

Infusions

Infusions and decoctions are two of the simplest and most rewarding types of herbal preparations available to you in your home kitchen. Both involve water, plant material, and heat. Together, the three humble elements alchemize into potent high-nutrient potions. Boiling, simmering, and slowly soaking herbs in warm water extract healing compounds with time and care. Water is a universal solvent and an infusion is, simply put, an herbal tea made from steeping plants in water. Herb infusions are among the simplest and most ancient forms of herbal extracts.

Herbal infusions are made by steeping herbs (leaves, flowers, stems) in hot water for as little as three minutes or as long as twenty minutes—and in some cases even longer. Infusions are used for plant materials like leaves, flowers, and stems or aerial parts. But the types of infusion vary widely. You can make an infusion from fresh herbs, dried herbs, and even powdered herbs. You can make a quick infusion in boiling water, or a long cold-water infusion under the light of the sun or the moon. Roots, seeds, and bark are better extracted in hot water or through a decoction. Fresh garden herbs like nettle and red raspberry leaf, along with tender flower blooms, lend themselves well to sun infusion. Herbs like mugwort and sage are well extracted in a moon infusion.

Infusions are easy to work into your daily routine. With a few herbs at hand, herbal teas can be customized and personalized to reflect your current needs. It is recommended you work with fresh garden herbs when possible or dried whole herbs bought at the herb store or online from a trusted source, as opposed to working with herbal tea bags or boxed tisanes.

When making infusions, I recommend avoiding tea bags for a few reasons. First, herbs in tea bags are often stale, as they may have been powdered and packaged a long time ago. The freshness of the herb is gone, along with its healing benefits. What's more, herbal tea bags often combine different plant parts that require different extraction methods. For instance, a tea bag blend may include both leaf and root parts. Most herb roots require a longer steeping method and won't release their therapeutic compounds through a five-minute soak in a cup of hot water.

If you enjoy tea bags, upgrading to a loose-leaf herbal infusion is a big yet simple step toward reclaiming a more embodied herbal practice. You'll get to craft custom blends and experience a wide spectrum of taste and feel as you watch loose herbs dance and unfurl in the water as they steep, coloring your infusion with a hue that no tea bag can rival and filling your herbal kitchen with an enticing and grounding aroma.

When you are working with herbal infusions, you might think that you need a higher ratio of dried plant versus fresh plant, but the opposite is true: a dried herb is more concentrated than its fresh counterpart because of decreased water content, so you actually need less plant material. Some herbs taste awful—skip the herbal tea for them and enjoy them in other ways.

Different solvents (such as water, alcohol, oil, glycerin, wine, or honey) extract different herbal compounds. An herbal infusion in water allows for a good extraction of vitamins and minerals along with polysaccharides, mucilage, tannins, and starches when compared with other solvents. Hot infusions also draw out enzymes and aromatic volatile oils. When used fresh, store your infusion in the fridge and consume it within one to three days. You can pour strong herbal tea into the bath for a healing herbal soak, or freeze your infusions into ice cubes to enjoy with sparkling water and tasty cocktails or thrown into smoothies.

Decoctions

Decoctions are quite similar to infusions except that they involve a longer, hotter steeping period in simmering water. Whereas herbal infusions are made by steeping herbs in hot water for as little as three minutes or as long as twenty minutes, and in some cases up to sixty minutes, herbal decoctions are simmered for up to thirty minutes, and in some cases for hours.

A decoction is made by boiling the plant material in water, and an infusion is made by steeping the plant material in hot water that has just been boiled. Decoctions are often more concentrated than infusions due to their longer simmer time. Use decoctions when dealing with harder-to-extract material such as wood-hard mushrooms, seeds and dried berries, barks, and stiff roots. The longer steeping period allows for the extraction of harder-to-reach plant material.

You can turn decoctions into syrups. Decoctions, like infusions, make great additions to bath water. They can also be frozen into ice cube trays for later use. Whereas herbal teas will last for one to three days in the refrigerator, decoctions typically last a bit longer; they keep fresh for four to five days.

Contraindications for Infusions and Decoctions

Avoid using herbs with unpleasant tastes in infusions and decoctions because they will reduce compliance. Compliance is the concept of herbal remedies being ingested and used regularly. If the herbal remedies taste bad, you and your clients won't enjoy taking them. Therefore, folks are more likely to abandon the protocol or to not follow it regularly. This will in turn affect results. In some cases, adjuvant herbs can be added to jazz up taste, color, and aroma. Common adjuvant herbs include fennel seeds, ginger, hibiscus, peppermint, and licorice. For best results, design herbal-tea experiences that taste and feel delicious and delightful.

Drying

Drying your herbs is one of the best and most reliable preservation methods. The vast majority of medicinal herbs retain their active compounds when dried. The main purpose of drying herbs is to have access to them all year long and outside their growing season. You can dry them in a dehydrator on low setting, in a stackable drying rack with screening, or tied in bundles and hung in the air. For best results, your drying place should be dark and dry, as both light and moisture will negatively impact the drying process.

When drying leaves and flowers, it is best to leave them whole but removed from the stem, because the stem contains more moisture. Roots should be cleaned and sliced before drying because they tend to become rock-hard as they dry and nearly impossible to slice. The same is true of many polypore mushrooms. Dried herbs are used for making infusions, decoctions, powders, syrups, herbal wines, herbal baths, oils, salves, and liquid extracts. Dried leaves and flowers can keep for as long as one year once dried, provided they are stored well. Roots, barks, mushrooms, and seeds can keep for as long as two to three years. Store your dried herbs in a glass jar and away from sunlight.

Powders

Powders are processed from dried herbs and are highly concentrated. Powders are enjoyed as a base ingredient for food and drink recipes and are used to make infusions, elixirs, bliss balls, syrups, herbal wines, herbal baths, oils, salves, and tinctures (and anything else your mind dreams up). Using herbs in their powder form is a potent and therapeutic use of plants as medicine. Tonic herbs are used in this way in the ancient medicine systems of Ayurveda and Traditional Chinese Medicine.

Compared with other herbal preparations like tinctures and liquid extracts, powdered herbs have no alcohol content, are highly bioavailable, and retain a high level of active constituents when used correctly. Since the whole plant part is dried and ground into a powder, there is none of the waste associated with extracts where the plant material is discarded after extraction. With plant powders, there is no room to hide a low-quality product. Bright color, taste, and freshness are all indicators of a plant powder rich in healing compounds. As such, they are one of the least shelf-stable herbal preparations and should be used within six to twelve months for best benefits. Plant powders can be added to carriers like warm plant milks or honey for an instant and convenient elixir.

Herb powders are typically not made from scratch at home and rather are bought from herb suppliers because grinding herbs into a fine and smooth powder requires the right milling equipment. Powders made at home in a coffee grinder or with other kitchen tools tend to be gritty with small herb chunks of uneven size that don't compare with the silky smooth experience of a fine herb powder.

Syrups

Syrups are tasty liquid extracts made from an herbal decoction and preserved with glycerin, honey, maple syrup, or other sweeteners like cane sugar. A small part of alcohol or alcohol-based herbal tincture can be added to a syrup to lengthen its shelf life. Herbal syrups are taken by the spoonful, added to a cup of steaming herbal tea, or mixed with sparkling water, kombucha, or cocktails. Syrups can be made into infinite variations. First, it starts with an herbal infusion or decoction, which are made from fresh herbs, dried herbs, powdered herbs, or a combination of the three. After straining the resulting tea, it is placed back on the stovetop to reduce by about half its volume. For herbal syrup making, a volume of 1-to-1 tea to sweetener is often used, or 2-to-1 if alcohol is added for preservation.

Any herb in the intimate materia medica that is a good indication for you based on your constitution, health conditions, and personal wellness goals can be made into a syrup and enjoyed regularly. There is no limit to the flavors that can be conjured in an herbal syrup. From forest mushrooms to circulation-enhancing rosemary to heart-warming aromatics like ginger and cardamom, syrups present a formula where delicious flavors are a part of the medicine.

Herbal Wines

Herbal wines, meads, ciders, beers, and liqueurs have a long and rich history of use. Medicinal herbal wines have been found in ancient Egypt and were widely used in Traditional Chinese Medicine for enriching restoration, while herb and wine formulas maintained a recognized status by the *U.S. Pharmacopeia* in the early 20th century.[2]

Volatile aromatic compounds in digestive and liver-supporting herbs are distinctly suitable to wine and other alcohol-based solvents, which are fast-acting because alcohol enters our bloodstream quickly. Herbal wines stimulate the nervous and circulatory systems, offer a warming boost to digestion, and raise the spirits. Herbal wines are made with fresh, dried, or powdered herbs. The combinations are endlessly varied and offer room for creativity and experimentation. A sip of handcrafted herbal wine shared with a lover sets the tone for a sensual mood, while the steeped medicinal herbs help awaken the body and warm the heart.

Homebrewers and crafters will enjoy making herbal wines from scratch by making their own ferments and adding herbs throughout the various stages of brewing and aging. But it is just as beneficial from an herbal standpoint to simply add herbs to infuse in ready-made wine, cider, mead, and liqueur. Choose herbs and herb profiles that have a pleasant taste and that blend well together. Start with small batches until you refine the blends that suit your palate best. Fennel seeds, schisandra berries, hibiscus, cacao nibs, orange peels, damiana, ginger, and rose all make delicious herbal wine pairings.

Herbal Baths and Soaks

There's something deeply soothing and healing about soaking in a large tub full of herbal tea made to fit the day's needs. Whether to nourish and revitalize, shift emotional states, or spark a sensual mood, therapeutic herbal baths are tailored to meet your needs. Herbs like milky oats, damiana, tulsi, rose, and rosemary make pleasurable and therapeutic additions to an herbal bath. The pores of the skin absorb the herbal benefits like thousands of tiny mouths, while the whole neurology of the person shifts from the combination of herbal medicine and hydrotherapy.

Nervous system conditions such as stress, burnout, and depression all have a strong affinity with a protocol of herbal baths. Herbal soaks are available to anyone with access to a tub and a large casserole pot to steep tea in. My favorite method for herbal baths is to bring a large pot of water to a boil, add a few handfuls of dried herbs like milky oats, damiana, tulsi, rose, and rosemary, cover, and let steep for fifteen to thirty minutes before straining. Fill a bathtub with warm water and add the herbal tea. You can steep the same herbs in the pot several times in order to get the most healing compounds out of them.

Oils and Salves

In the context of herbalism for sexual and reproductive health, oils and salves are herbal preparations meant for external use on the skin as well as over and in the genitals (like with herbal oil-based lubes). Certain herbs such as calendula, cleavers, and plantain lend themselves especially well to oil infusion because their constituents are oil-soluble and their properties as emollients make them great external remedies to be applied on the skin or the genitals. To make an herbal oil, place herbs and oil together in a jar in a ratio of 1-to-2 or 1-to-5 (1 part herb to 2 parts oil and up to 5 parts oil). Let infuse in a cool dark place for two to four weeks, strain, and bottle.

Infused herbal oils are the base for making salves. To make an herbal salve, add beeswax to an herbal oil and warm to melt together and combine. The salve will harden as it cools. Olive oil is a good solvent for herbal extractions, but oils like jojoba, sunflower, avocado, fractionated coconut, and others may be used as well. Herbal oils and salves make great massage oils and oil-based lubricants. Herbal oils keep for one to two years while herbal salves made from herbal oils will keep for three to five years, thanks to the preservative quality of beeswax.

Liquid Extracts (Tinctures)

Liquid extracts, also commonly called tinctures, may be the herbal remedy of our time because they are fast-acting and convenient to use, which suits busy lifestyles well. Liquid extracts are made with a variety of solvents. The most commonly used solvent is alcohol, but vinegar, honey, and glycerin are other possible options for tincturing herbs. Herbal tinctures in alcohol maintain their potency for up to ten years, making them one of the most desirable and ecological herbal preparations. The long shelf life of tinctures reduces the waste associated with dried herbs and herb powders, which lose their potency faster.

Because alcohol extracts herbal compounds so well, making them quite concentrated, less plant matter is needed per dose than with other herbal preparations like infusions or decoctions. Compared with other solvents, alcohol extracts alkaloids, glycosides, resins, and essential oils. It does not extract minerals or mucilage. Tinctures are commonly made from grain alcohol. At home, however, it's possible to use a variety of alcohols that may suit certain herbs best. Possible pairings include ginger and rum, damiana and tequila, and hibiscus and mezcal. For blended alcohol extracts, replace half the alcohol with molasses, maple syrup, or honey. Organic and locally made alcohols and sweeteners may be available based on where you live.

Herbal Chocolates

Is there a better, more satisfying way to engage with medicinal herbs than through the medium of chocolate? The handcrafted chocolate revolution is underway, and herbs and cacao make the perfect match. As a healing agent, natural cacao acts as a potent medicinal vessel for herbs and plant extracts. Herbal chocolates can be eaten as small treats, drunk in the form of hot chocolate, drizzled over food, or turned into various delectable concoctions.

One of my favorite ways to enjoy herbal chocolates is in the form of a chocolate bark, where a liquid cacao base is poured over a sheet and left to solidify at room temperature, laden with a colorful layer of herb powders, flower petals, and pollen. For a chocolate bar, a large quantity of medicinal herb powders can seamlessly be added into your cacao mixture before pouring into a mold. Chocolate cups can be filled with a blend of coconut butter, honey, and herbal powders mixed with liquid extracts. The possibilities are endless.

How to Store Herbs and Herbal Preparations

When working with fresh herbs from the garden or the wild, a few considerations apply. Fresh herbs need to be processed before they spoil—this happens very quickly with leaves and flowers. Herb processing includes separating wilted leaves from vibrant ones and removing tiny insects and various plant material from your desired plant parts. As a rule of thumb, it's recommended that whenever you go out foraging, allow for at least an hour of processing for each hour of foraging. If you don't have time to process afterward, your foraged plant material will go to waste.

Once your plant parts have been thoroughly cleaned and processed, extraction can begin: drying, infusing, or steeping in oil, alcohol, or other solvents. Once extracted, herb preparations are labeled and properly stored. Dried herbs and herb powders should be kept in clean glass jars away from direct heat and sunlight and replaced every year. One of the most important rules to stick to when you make herbal preparations is to label everything. Keep labels on hand and use them. Write down the herb, herb part, extraction method, ingredients used, and date. You might want to dedicate a cupboard or cabinet to your herbs and intimate herbal pharmacy.

What to Look for When Buying and Using Herbs

As herbal medicine gains popularity, it becomes easier to find high-quality herbs and herbal products to purchase. On a personal level, you want to make sure the herbs you purchase are really what they are supposed to be. There have been many instances of medicinal herbs sold that turned out to be a different species from what was advertised or had been diluted with other unrelated herbs or substances altogether. For example, I know a couple of spice importers who have seen crushed orange-colored bricks sold as turmeric powder. The surest way to avoid this is to grow and harvest herbs yourself or buy herbs from a reputable supplier.

When it comes to buying herbal products, it is crucial to buy products where every ingredient is listed on the label. Avoid purchasing "mystery blends" or products labeled with little care. Herbal products should clearly list herb ratios, the herb parts used, the menstruum used, the extraction method, and the best-before date. Most reputable herbal product providers list herbs in binomial nomenclature to avoid confusion, which means you'll find the Latin herb name rather than the common name listed on the label. Consult an herbalist before buying or using herbal products. Talk about your current health conditions, medications, allergies, and other relevant health information.

On a broader level, buying and using medicinal herb products involve a thorough search into the growing practices and sustainability of the herbs we use. Many popular medicinal herbs are at risk of extinction as a result of overharvesting, while others may require specific growing conditions in which to thrive. Medicinal plants are valuable sources of herbal products, and they are disappearing at high speed. But sourcing high-quality, vibrant, organically grown medicinal herbs is now easier than ever.

Organic farming, along with biodynamic farming and regenerative agriculture, creates integrated, humane, and environmentally and economically sustainable production systems for medicinal plants. Organically grown medicinal herbs help maintain ecological balance and enhance soil health. Organic farming of medicinal plants is becoming increasingly important in the long-term development and sustainability of herbalism, along with small-scale home gardens and community gardens.

Small-scale gardeners and growers often forgo the official organic certification, which can be costly and inaccessible to tiny farm operations. Many of my farming friends haven't sought to be organic-certified—instead, they invite folks to visit the farm and see the holistic land and naturally nurtured plants for themselves. The community-based beyond-organic movement is taking shape among herbalists young and old and encourages you to get to know your herb farmer, participate in apothecary co-ops and community-supported agriculture (CSA) programs, and support herb farms near and far.

Herbal Troubleshooting

Despite our best planning and intentions, sometimes herbs or an herbal protocol don't deliver the results we had hoped for. There's an array of possible reasons for this, but here are a few of the most common reasons we encounter in herbal practice why herbs might not work. The following reasons are in four categories: herb quality, formula quality, individual reasons, and collective reasons.

Herb Quality Troubleshooting

- The herbs used are old or expired and no longer vibrant. Their active compounds are diminished.

- The wrong herb part was used.

- The herb part was harvested at the wrong moment in the growth cycle.

- The herbs were grown in or harvested from a polluted or contaminated environment.

- The herbs were grown using pesticides or herbicides.

- The herbs were grown in depleted soil and are low in nutritional value.

- The herb is not really what it says on the label. It's a different species or genus. In the case of rare and pricey herbs, there are often substitutions made to cut costs, which means the buyer gets a lower-quality product.

When it comes to herb quality and the effectiveness of herbs and herbal protocols, there are simple solutions. First of all, buy herbs from reputable sources. Be willing to pay more for a higher-quality product, or grow and process the herbs yourself. Small-scale local herbalists are your best source of quality herbs. Buy local when possible and encourage farmers who practice organic or biodynamic principles. Keep your home apothecary well organized, label everything, and keep track of herb expiration dates. Toss old herbs in the compost. If you're not yet proficient and experienced at herbal harvesting and processing, and aren't sure which herb part to use for a specific purpose, work with trained herbalists to assist you through that process.

Formula Quality Troubleshooting

- The wrong preparation method was used for the herb part and formula goal.

- Extraction time was too short.

- The wrong solvent was used for the desired extraction.

- The quantity of plant material used in an herbal preparation was insufficient.

- Herbs with opposing actions were used in the same formula, thus reducing the other's desired action.

- There are too many herbs in a single formula, or the herbs chosen don't work well together.

Herbal preparations are an art and science. You don't need any special equipment, but knowing your herbs well is a must. Start slow and get to know only a small handful of herbs at a time. Start formulating only when you feel confident that you know an herb well. Many herbal apprentices today are in a rush to use hundreds of herbs before they're ready, which can result in clumsy formulas and extractions. The truth is, it's not the number of herbs you know that make you a great herbalist. Rather, it's the intimate relationship you can build with herbs that will change the way you formulate and work with them.

As in life, it can be more rewarding and valuable to maintain a small handful of close, precious, and deep friendships rather than a hundred somewhat superficial ones. The economy of scale mentality has pervaded our minds and relationships, but more is not always better. Like the slow food and slow sex movements, we need a slow herb movement too. It may seem radical in our fast-paced world, but many old-time herbalists recommend spending one month with a single herb. Some herbal apprenticeships follow an entire one-year journey with a single herb. Imagine getting to know a single herb that well. How might that change your formulas?

Individual Reasons Troubleshooting

- The person taking the herb or herbal protocol doesn't take the right dosage.

- The person takes the remedies inconsistently.

- The person stops the protocol too early, or as soon as they start to feel better.

- The person doesn't change their diet or lifestyle, which may have caused their symptoms or health imbalances in the first place.

- The person doesn't actually want to get better. There may be other unconscious attachments to poor health or persistent symptoms.

- The person is taking the herbal remedies in excess, which taxes the body.

- The person is using an herb that covers the symptoms rather than addressing the root cause of the problem.

- The person is using a stimulating herb that furthers depletion, which impedes healing.

- The person doesn't assimilate nutrients as a result of poor digestion, thus affecting the efficiency of herbs and formulas.

Collective Reasons Troubleshooting

When herbs and herbal protocols fail to deliver the hoped-for results, sometimes it's not because there's something wrong with the herb, with the formula, or with the way a person follows the protocol. It can be tempting to zoom in to precise individual reasons why herbs don't work, but it's important at times to zoom out too. We live within a larger context of society, environment, and culture that all affect sexual health and wellness.

Sometimes herbs and herbal protocols are no match for the harmful impacts of poverty, pollution, sexism, racism, and other oppressions. There is a lot of inequality in the world, and humble herbs, as amazing and generous as they are, are simply not magic bullets. That doesn't mean you shouldn't bother taking them, though. When we stop expecting that herbs are a panacea and that working with herbs will fix all of our problems and the problems of the world, we can start to build a real relationship with them and welcome them as true herbal allies in our lives.

5

Sexual and Reproductive Health

Introduction to Sexual and Reproductive Health

Sexual and reproductive health is our birthright. Sex, intimacy, fertility, and sexual and reproductive wellness are an essential part of healthy living. In today's world, it's also something we have to actively protect, reclaim, encourage, and celebrate. Many modern challenges collide to negatively impact and harm sexual pleasure and reproductive function. Hormonal imbalances are on a steep rise while fertility levels continue to plummet to a dangerous low. The consequences of poor nutrition, environmental pollutants and everyday toxins, systemic disempowerment as it relates to preventative health and self-care, and high-stress lifestyles all show up in ways that can affect libido, fertility, and the ability to enjoy an embodied sensual life.

Medicinal herbs have a beneficial impact on hormones, physiological function, and body chemistry. The adoption of herbal remedies and practices supports and sustains sexual and reproductive wellness. Along with herbal medicine, essential knowledge to reclaim includes body literacy and a basic understanding of sexual and reproductive anatomy, physiology, and hormones.

Sexual and Reproductive Anatomy and Physiology

The field of sexual and reproductive health is one where gendered language is commonly used. But it's important to note that anatomy and physiology do not define gender. Many of us involved with herbalism today will benefit from a better understanding of the gender spectrum that goes beyond the binary of male or female. For health practitioners, gender inclusivity is not only beneficial but truly essential. It must be learned so that we can better serve our transgender, genderqueer, and gender-nonbinary clients and community members.

In some instances, the use of gender-neutral terms is easy to adopt. Words like *parent* instead of *mother* and *father, partner* instead of *girlfriend* and *boyfriend* or *wife* and *husband,* and *child* instead of *daughter* and *son* are all examples of appropriate gender-neutral and inclusive terms. However, as practitioners, we have not yet come up with language for discussing anatomical systems that have been historically discussed in gendered terms.

For that reason, and for the sake of simplicity, when it comes to discussing anatomy and physiology in these pages, I will at times refer to the vagina, uterus, and related sexual organs as "women's bodies," "female sexual organs," and other such gendered assumptions. The same goes for penises and prostates, which I will at times refer to as "men's bodies," "male sexual organs," and "the male reproductive system."

Female Sexual and Reproductive Anatomy

Clitoris: The part of the clitoris we are familiar with is about the size of a pea and sits just above the urethral opening. This is the glans clitoris and represents only about 10 percent of the total surface of the clitoris. Like the tip of an iceberg, the glans clitoris connects to the clitoris hidden below the surface, encircling the vagina and extending into the pelvis.

Is Everything You've Learned About the Clit Wrong?

French researcher and science sociologist Odile Fillod has shaken up the world of women's anatomy with her recent 3-D-printed anatomically correct clitoris. It looks nothing like what sex ed taught you. In 2019, she succeeded in having four of the largest publishers of French educational manuals revise their anatomy books in order to dispel the myth that the clit is a "little button." This little button is in fact just the glans, or the tip of the clitoral iceberg.

Labia: The labia comprise the labia majora, the outer lips, and labia minora, the small inner lips. Together they protect the clitoris, urethral opening, and vaginal opening. They also hold two pairs of small secretory glands that supply lubrication and alkaline fluids that help protect the vulva and vagina against infection. Every set of labia is unique.

Vulva: The clitoris and labia together make the vulva.

Vagina: The vagina connects the vulva (external) with the internal organs (cervix, uterus, and ovaries). It's a muscular tube that ranges four to seven inches long. The vagina also serves as a birth canal during birthing. The vagina possesses many nerve endings for pleasurable stimulation and houses the G-spot.

Cervix: Located at the upper end of the vagina, the cervix leads to the uterus. The cervix changes shape, texture, and location throughout the menstrual cycle. For instance, it's softer and higher up the vagina during ovulation, and harder and lower down the vagina during menstruation.

Uterus: About the size and shape of a pear, the uterus is connected to the fallopian tubes, which deliver the egg released every month by one of the two ovaries. The wall of the uterus is divided into three main layers: the perimetrium, myometrium, and the endometrium.

Changes in uterine function, such as menstruation, are regulated by hormones secreted by the hypothalamus, the pituitary gland, and the ovaries. This feedback loop is called the HPO axis, or HPAO to include the adrenal glands, and involves neurotransmitters, endorphins, luteinizing hormone, follicle-stimulating hormone, estrogen, progestins, and androgens.

Ovaries: The ovaries are small oblong organs located in the pelvis and that rest on either side of the uterus. The orifice of the fallopian tube is located just above each ovary, close but not in direct contact, with the tube leading to the uterus. The ovaries produce eggs. What's more, they also play an essential role in the hormonal system, helping produce estrogen, progesterone, and androgens.

Important hormones involved in female sexual and reproductive function include the steroidal hormones estrogen, progesterone, and testosterone along with the glycoprotein hormones follicle-stimulating hormone (FSH) and luteinizing hormone (LH). FSH and LH are released by the pituitary gland and regulate the entire ovarian cycle via feedback loops governed by varying levels of estrogen, progesterone, and inhibin. Luteinizing hormone triggers ovulation while FSH brings the follicle to maturation.

Male Sexual and Reproductive Anatomy

Penis: The penis is made of the glans, or tip of the penis, along with the shaft, which contains the urethra, the foreskin, and the frenulum.

Scrotum: The scrotum holds the testicles and keeps them at the right temperature by adjusting its position closer to the body when it's cold and farther away from the body when it's warm.

Testicles: The testicles are two ball-like glands that produce sperm and hormones like testosterone. Testicles are held in the scrotum.

Seminal vesicles: Located below the bladder, the seminal vesicles are two small organs responsible for producing semen, the fluid that carries sperm during ejaculation. The vas deferens carries sperm from the epididymis, the tube where sperm matures, to the seminal vesicles.

Prostate gland: Surrounding the neck of the bladder and urethra in the shape of a donut, the prostate gland is the size of a walnut and secretes seminal fluid, an alkaline fluid that forms part of semen. It also helps propel semen from the penis. The prostate is pleasurable to the touch (via the anus) and is known as the male G-spot.

Important hormones involved in male sexual and reproductive function include FSH, LH, and testosterone. FSH is necessary for sperm production and triggers the testes into secreting androgen binding protein (ABP), which brings the cells to be more receptive to testosterone. Luteinizing hormone, on the other hand, stimulates the production of testosterone, followed by spermatogenesis. Testosterone helps regulate sex drive and libido while building muscle mass and strength.

A Holistic Understanding of Sexuality, Fertility, and Cycles

Vaginas and penises are not the only sexual organs. Orgasm actually happens in the brain.[1] Orgasm can happen without any stimulation or sensation in particular nerves, which is great news for folks with spinal cord injuries, and also explains why we can enjoy orgasm in our dreams. The brain is a sexual powerhouse and controls the sexual response, influenced by sexual fantasies, images, and sensual moods. The skin is also a sexual organ, with millions of sensitive nerves that respond to touch and spark relaxation, arousal, and stimulation.

What about sex hormones? From a hormonal perspective, all human bodies produce the same steroidal hormones, but in differing quantities. This includes estrogens, progesterone, testosterone, and other androgens. And all human bodies produce the same glycoprotein hormones: LH and FSH. Clinical herbalist Kara Sigler points out that these hormones act in similar ways, though with slightly different outcomes, based on the body's gamete makeup and steroidal hormone proclivity.[2]

The endocrine system signals the release of steroid hormones from the pituitary gland (LH, FSH, oxytocin, prolactin), ovaries (estrogen, progesterone), and testes (testosterone). But physiological and psychological stress overload can affect the process and lead to endocrine dysregulation. This includes the impact of pollution, the presence of endocrine disruptors in consumer products, intersecting structural oppressions such as racism and sexism, as well as low-nutrient diets, overwork, and chronic inflammation.

Alterations in overall endocrine function alter sexual health and fertility through similar channels for folks of all genders. While standard approaches focus on psychological and physiological treatment, a truly integrated, holistic herbal approach rather targets underlying dysregulation stemming from a variety of personal, interpersonal, systemic, and environmental factors.

The physiology of arousal, sex, and fertility involves a rich web of interactions between sexual and reproductive organs, the nervous system, the brain, hormonal feedback loops, and the release of neurotransmitters. Like an intricate dance, the flow of sexual response includes excitement (desire and arousal), plateau, orgasm, and resolution. Dopamine sparks arousal, followed by oxytocin. Androgens activate nitric oxide pathways and further facilitate dopamine release. The parasympathetic nervous system delivers blood flow to the genitals and swells erectile tissue, engorging the clitoris and the penis as well as the nipples.

The hormones and organs involved in the sexual response are influenced positively with medicinal herbs. The herbs included in our materia medica for intimate herbalism bring benefits to the full-spectrum experience of sexual health, fertility, and hormonal balance. They include nervine herbs, adaptogen herbs, tonic herbs, nutritive herbs, and hormonal herbs, a group of herbs I call full-spectrum aphrodisiacs.

6

Intimate Health Conditions

Introduction to Health Conditions

In the following sections, common health conditions relevant to intimate health and the sexual and reproductive organs are listed and explored along with clear guidelines for herbal protocols. Where applicable, modern scientific advances relevant to herbs have been included. Some herbs have many scientific validations to back them up, while other herbs are used by herbalists and known to work, albeit without much scientific cred compiled yet on their behalf. As such, you'll notice that some herbs listed in the following pages have studies and data associated with their use, while other herbs are explained in simpler terms based on tradition and herb lore.

The dosage and recommended applications of each herb for specific conditions have been left voluntarily open-ended, as each person may react to herbs and dosages differently. For herbalists, the protocols and herbs listed will offer helpful starting points and leads. For those who don't practice herbalism, it's recommended that you work with an herbalist to help you on your path to sexual and reproductive healing along with these protocols.

Conditions run the spectrum from short-term and acute to long-term and chronic. Some are a direct reaction to specific life events, while others may be metabolic and systemic with causes that are broader and harder to pinpoint. Still other conditions aren't imbalances at all but rather necessary life stages or normal processes that may still carry with them symptoms that folks wish to address with herbs and herbal protocols for relief and comfort.

I've witnessed full recoveries from an array of health conditions as a direct result of using the right plants in the right dosage at the right time. When used preventively, herbs protect and guard against the development of illness or imbalances. Still at other times, herbal protocols may work to soothe symptoms and keep the body in a place of harmony even in the context of an ongoing health crisis that herbs alone can't treat or reverse. No matter where you are on your sexual and reproductive health journey, herbs can help. In this chapter, we explore all the ways we can ally with medicinal herbs to build sexual and reproductive wellness, optimal fertility levels, and balanced cycles, naturally.

Breast Health

Women's breasts are made of fatty tissue, veins, arteries, mammary glands, connective tissue, lymph vessels, and lymph nodes, along with the nerves responsible for the whole-body sensation felt when breasts are touched in pleasurable ways.

Each breast is made of many sections called lobes that are shaped and positioned like the petals of a daisy. Because breasts are mostly made of fat, they don't benefit from as much blood flow as other parts of the body. Muscles lie under each breast and over the ribs, with no muscles present in the breast itself. As fatty tissue, breasts can act as a toxin collection and storage area where harmful pollutants may accumulate.

Recent studies have demonstrated the presence of toxic metals like mercury and aluminum in breast tissue.[1] Breasts are like sponges, soaking up fat-soluble chemicals, and are particularly vulnerable to carcinogens. Common breast conditions include cysts and lumps, breast cancer, and sore and cracked nipples. But breasts respond well to lifestyle choices and healing medicinal herbs. Even in a toxic world, it's possible to treat your breasts well.

To sustain and promote healthy breasts, eat a nutrient-rich diet and choose organically grown foods as much as possible to reduce exposure to pesticides, herbicides, and other contaminants such as lipophilic toxins that accumulate in fatty tissues in the breasts. These fat-soluble endocrine-disrupting toxins have been found in breast milk as a result of exposure in the diet and conventional foodways. Aside from foods, practice wholesome rest and relaxation to support breast health. Give yourself a gentle breast massage with herbal oils on a regular basis. These are simple but powerful and reliable guidelines for healthy breasts.

Despite following the healthiest diet and lifestyle, some outside factors harmful to breast health are hard to avoid individually and collectively. This includes the negative effects of environmental pollution and the widespread presence of xenoestrogens, a group of endocrine disruptors that specifically have estrogen-like effects, found in countless consumer items like plastic containers and body-care products. When breast conditions happen, herbs can help.

Breast health is affected by the impacts of sexism, racism, and other intersecting oppressions. For example, a lack of risk assessment, prevention, and early detection along with low inclusion in clinical trials contributes to a much higher mortality rate from breast cancer in Black communities when compared with that of White communities. Indigenous women are more likely to be diagnosed with breast cancer at a later stage (stage 2 or higher) than nonindigenous women.

From a preventative herbal health and self-care approach, you can support breast health with nutritive herbs to keep the whole body optimally nourished and well equipped to fight off imbalances. Add alterative herbs to assist with daily cleansing and the elimination of toxins, and lymphatic herbs to keep lymph flowing and to prevent stagnation. Nervine herbs relieve stress and exhaustion, lift mood, and support the health of the nervous system.

Nutritive herbs are herbal superfoods and provide a wealth of highly bioavailable nutrients. Nettle (calcium, iron, potassium, chlorophyll, vitamins), milky oats (vitamin C, carotene, phosphorus, potassium, iron, B vitamins), red raspberry leaf (vitamin C, carotene, iron, magnesium, calcium, potassium), dandelion (folate, calcium, magnesium, potassium, iron, vitamin C, carotene), and red clover (calcium, chromium, magnesium, niacin, phosphorus, potassium, thiamine, vitamin C) are potent nutritive herbs that support breast health via enhanced nutrient stores.

Alterative herbs support the metabolism and improve the body's ability to eliminate waste through the major eliminatory organs (lungs, lymph, skin, kidneys, liver, and bowels). Better detoxification and elimination supported by alterative herbs improve the body's abilities to heal and function in a healthy manner. In other words, alterative herbs are gentle and efficient detoxifiers. Alterative herbs beneficial for breast health include cleavers, calendula, red clover, dandelion, and nettle.

Lymphatic herbs help move lymph and can increase lymphatic flow by moving fluid and protein away from inflamed areas. As a result, fresh lymph rich in oxygen and nutrients needed for tissue repair floods in, preventing congestion and swelling. Lymph contains lymphocytes, white blood cells that fight infections and defend against diseases like cancer. Calendula, cleavers, and red clover are lymphatic herbs used for breast health.

Nervine herbs are beneficial every day, but especially so in the context of illness or imbalance when emotions run high. Fear, anxiety, pain, discomfort, and insomnia can occur alongside breast conditions. Stress compounds health imbalances by provoking the body into a state of hyper alert and the release of stress hormones that can further increase symptoms in both physical and psychosomatic ways. Nervine herbs beneficial in the context of breast health include milky oats, passionflower, valerian, and California poppy.

Breast Cysts

This condition is also called fibrocystic breast and can make breasts feel tender and lumpy. Many health practitioners disagree with the term *fibrocystic breast disease* that has been used in the past to describe this condition because it pathologizes what can be entirely normal cyclic changes in breast tissue. Another common name for the condition is cyclical mastalgia. Breast cysts are characterized by breast pain, swelling, and noncancerous lumps. While any lumps in the breast should be checked by a doctor to rule out the potential for breast cancer, the condition of breast cysts is considered to be uncomfortable but not particularly dangerous.

Many health practitioners believe that breast cysts are influenced by hormonal fluctuations and estrogen and progesterone imbalance. The fact that symptoms associated with breast cysts often increase monthly right before menstruation and disappear altogether at the onset of menopause supports the view that breast cysts are related to reproductive hormones, especially estrogen excess. From an herbal perspective, much help is found with herbs. Nutritive, alterative, and lymphatic herbs decongest the lymphatic system and the liver, while nervine herbs settle emotional symptoms and balance stress. Medicinal herbs with a strong affinity for support with breast cysts include red clover, cleavers, and dandelion.

Red clover is an alterative herb for blood purification with a specific affinity for the lymphatic tissues. It is a beneficial nutritive tonic and beneficial source of isoflavones. The mildly estrogenic activity of red clover isoflavones is many times less active than the activity of steroidal estrogen. One study in premenopausal women showed an antiestrogenic effect from red clover by relieving breast pain associated with fibrocystic breast pain.[2]

Another trial on the long-term effect of a red clover–derived isoflavone supplement taken daily for one year concluded that, unlike conventional hormone replacement therapy, the red clover supplement did not increase mammographic breast density.[3] High mammographic breast density is a known risk factor for breast cancer. Even women with a family history of breast cancer have been shown to safely consume red clover isoflavones in a three-year study.[4] Drink red clover as an infusion. Pair it with nettle and milky oats to enhance nutrition and calm the nervous system.

Cleavers is a lymphatic alterative herb. It cleanses excessive fluids from the body. Cleavers eases tender swollen breasts and shrinks cysts and lumps. Cleavers needs to be taken regularly over long periods of time in order to deliver its full desired effect. It is best used fresh or extracted fresh. Enjoy cleavers as an herbal tea during the warmer months, and harvest the fresh green and sticky plant to extract in the juicer to use for the rest of the year. The bright-green and chlorophyll-rich juice of cleavers can be stored in ice cube trays and kept frozen to add to smoothies, juices, and soups.

Dandelion offers therapeutic benefits for breast health. Both dandelion root and dandelion leaf provide nutrients and therapeutic properties. The leaf is bitter and nutrient-rich while the root is a liver tonic and cholagogue to increase the flow of bile and facilitate digestion. Herbal liver support from bitter herbs like dandelion enhances how the liver metabolizes steroid hormones. The liver is the primary site for estrogen clearance or estrogen metabolism. A compromised liver function can lead to a state of estrogen dominance that contributes to texture and density changes in the breast. Enjoy fresh dandelion leaf in salads and soups. Dandelion root can be taken in decoctions, liquid extracts, and capsules.

Breast Cancer

Breast cancer is the leading cause of cancer death among women worldwide. But current early detection methods allow breast cancer to be diagnosed at an early stage when treatment is more likely to be successful and to result in recovery. From a preventative perspective, many herbs possess anticancer properties.[5] Plant-based compounds for breast cancer prevention include alkaloids, phenol compounds, and monoterpenes. Turmeric, ginseng, milk thistle, and astragalus are examples of breast cancer–fighting herbs recognized by science and traditional use.

Turmeric is anticancer, anti-inflammatory, and antioxidant.[6] Curcumin, a polyphenol and one of the principal active components of turmeric, has therapeutic activities against breast cancer through multiple signaling pathways. Curcumin inhibits cell proliferation, promotes cell apoptosis (programmed cell death), prevents tumor angiogenesis and metastasis, and induces autophagy. Curcumin enhances the cytotoxicity effect of natural killer (NK) cells when these cells are cocultured with human breast cancer. For best results, take turmeric in the form of capsules.

Ginseng offers anticancer protection.[7] Ginsenoside is one of the main active ingredients in ginseng, and some polysaccharides and amino acids in ginseng also have pharmacological functions. Ginsenosides are triterpenoids and have anticancer activities. It also has a good effect in inhibiting breast cancer invasion and metastasis. In addition to its excellent anticancer properties, ginseng's immunomodulatory properties make it a good choice for the anticancer herbal pharmacy. Take ginseng as a liquid extract or in capsule form.

Milk thistle is a liver herb with anticancer activity that has been found useful against breast cancer.[8] Silibinin, one of the flavonoids isolated from milk thistle, displays various biological activities including antioxidative, antiproliferative, antibacterial, antifungal, neuroprotective, and antimetastatic activities. Silibinin has immunomodulatory and antitumor effects beneficial for breast cancer prevention. Milk thistle seed is commonly used as a tincture.

Astragalus is an adaptogen herb that can be used both preventively against breast cancer and also in conjunction with chemotherapy drugs.[9] Astragalus polysaccharides and astragaloside, important medicinal compounds in astragalus root, possess good immune and antiviral functions. Astragalus has attracted much attention because of its anticancer activity, with an obvious inhibitory effect on breast cancer. Astragalus can be taken as a single medicine and also used to synergistically enhance the efficacy of the chemotherapy drug cisplatin. Take astragalus in the form of a tincture or capsules.

A large and growing body of research indicates that environmental toxins released into the air, water, and soil are potent carcinogens. Exposure to harmful chemicals is ubiquitous today.[10] Plasticizers and other endocrine disruptors, pharmaceutical residue in drinking water, and chemical pesticides on food products all contribute to breast cancer risk; as other persistent organic pollutants (POPs) accumulate in soils, sediments, and in the air.

The extent and type of carcinogenic toxins folks are exposed to often depends on where they live and work. Poorer communities shoulder an unequal share of the burden of exposure to toxic materials. Studies have shown that while environmental conditions associated with low-income neighborhoods don't necessarily increase a woman's risk of being diagnosed with breast cancer, they do significantly increase a woman's risks of dying from it.[11]

Beyond prevention, herbs can help in the context of a breast cancer diagnosis as well. Medicinal herbs have important benefits when it comes to joint treatment in conjunction with chemotherapy, radiotherapy, surgery, and other methods of treatment for breast cancer.[12] Chemotherapy, radiotherapy, and surgery all carry significant side effects and health risks that medicinal herbs balance and mediate. Healing herbs lift the mental and emotional burdens associated with breast cancer and illness, such as depression, pain, fatigue, and psychoemotional distress.

Herbal remedies increase quality of life, improve immune function, decrease cytotoxicity to normal cells, support the body's natural defenses, balance moods, and otherwise bring care and natural nourishment to those undergoing breast cancer therapy. Medicinal herbs for breast cancer therapy include the adaptogenic herbs ashwagandha, dong quai, and *Panax ginseng*, along with the medicinal mushrooms codonopsis, turkey tail, and reishi.

An open-label, prospective, nonrandomized, comparative clinical study examined the use of ashwagandha root extract powder to relieve chemotherapy fatigue and improve quality of life in patients with breast cancer.[13] The study group took a dosage of 500 milligrams ashwagandha dry extract three times daily for six chemotherapy cycles.[14] The ashwagandha patients experienced less fatigue as well as better quality of life during chemotherapy than the control group.

Dong quai and *Panax ginseng* are used in herbal clinical practice for breast cancer treatment. Together, they decrease treatment-associated toxicity, psychosocial stress, and fatigue.

Reishi, codonopsis, and dong quai are used for their immunomodulating, anti-inflammatory, and wound-healing properties.[15] Preparations of turkey tail mushroom significantly improve appetite and alleviate weakness, vomiting, and pain while helping increase weight and stabilize white blood cell counts and natural killer cells. Turkey tail offers a 9 percent absolute reduction in the five-year mortality rate for cancer patients undergoing treatment.[16]

Polysaccharide-K (PSK), also known as krestin, is one of the active compounds found in turkey tail. It is a unique protein-bound polysaccharide and is used as a chemoimmunotherapy agent. PSK shows positive results in the adjuvant treatment of breast cancer and protects the patient from oxidative stress.

Reishi mushroom alleviates cancer-related fatigue in breast cancer patients undergoing chemotherapy and radiation treatment.[17] Patients who receive reishi report improved physical well-being, less fatigue, less anxiety and depression, and overall better quality of life. Kidney and liver function significantly improves with reishi intake, which helps lessen the risk of chemotherapy-induced renal dysfunction or liver damage.

The wide spectrum of biological effects reported for reishi in the prevention of chronic liver diseases makes it a viable adjuvant for hepatoprotection in breast cancer therapy. Among the active compounds present in reishi extracts, triterpenoids are one of the main components responsible for the pharmacological activities, including immunomodulatory, antioxidative, antimetastatic, and antitumor effects. In vitro and in vivo assays reveal that the mixtures of triterpenoids in reishi possess antiproliferative effects and induce apoptosis and cell-cycle arrest in cancer cells.[18] Medicinal mushrooms like turkey tail and reishi can be taken in powder form or in the form of capsules or liquid extract.

Sore and Cracked Nipples

Sore and cracked nipples are most often associated with breast-feeding, but other causes for nipple dryness, cracks, and irritation include eczema, contact dermatitis, and even running or jogging due to the nipples rubbing against fabric until they become raw and chafed. Medicinal herbs for sore and cracked nipples include wound-healing and emollient herbs calendula and plantain along with anti-inflammatory and skin-healing herbs comfrey and St. John's wort, applied topically as an herbal oil or salve.

Calendula flower is an anti-inflammatory, wound-healing, emollient, and antifungal herb. Calendula salve has a strong affinity for dry skin, eczema, and psoriasis, and for mom-and-baby care. Antifungal properties in calendula salve prevent nipple thrush.

Plantain leaf is a potent anti-inflammatory to reduce pain and swelling. It provides deep emollient hydration and repair. Plantain oil soothes inflamed tissues, itchiness, and redness. Applied over the breasts as a breast oil, plantain provides instant cooling and relief.

Comfrey leaf and root is an efficient wound healer that promotes cell regeneration. Always pair comfrey salve with an antimicrobial herb like calendula when applied on open cracks or wounds.

St. John's wort flower and aerial parts is an analgesic and anti-inflammatory herb. St. John's wort oil heals wounds and prevents scarring. Use it on red, cracked, burning, and painful nipples.

Breast Massage and Breast Oil

Breast massage with herbal oils builds an intimate knowledge of your breasts, their size and shape and cyclic fluctuations, while also enhancing circulation and preventing engorgement and tenderness. The practice of breast massage is thousands of years old and is rooted in self-care, wellness, and healing. Connected to sexuality and breast-feeding, breasts are a symbol of fertility and abundance.

Breast massage supports and heals breast tissue and promotes lymphatic flow. It enhances production of protective hormones like prolactin, oxytocin, and estrogen. Pair breast massage with healing herbs and herbal oils like dandelion, cleavers, chickweed, red clover, calendula, or yarrow. Here are some herbs beneficial for breast health when used as an infused massage oil.

Plantain oil relieves pain and swelling and is nourishing, healing, and profoundly anti-inflammatory.

St. John's wort oil repairs skin and nerve damage and supports the flow of lymph. It is a great ally during radiation treatment.

Yarrow oil is a circulatory tonic. It is antibacterial and relieves swelling and tenderness.

Lady's mantle oil eases lumps, swelling, and pain. Massaged over the breasts, it tones breast tissue.

Violet oil is healing to fibrocystic breasts, breast cancer, mastitis, and cysts.[19] It is a deeply soothing breast oil.

Cleavers oil decongests lymphatic tissue and enhances the flow of lymph. It possesses anti–breast cancer activity.[20]

Calendula oil is a healing lymphatic tonic. It acts as an alternative anti-inflammatory.

Contraception

The issue of contraception concerns people of reproductive age who wish to control when and how they conceive, along with those who wish to avoid conception and baby-making altogether. The goal of contraception is to prevent pregnancy while still enjoying penetrative sex, vaginal stimulation, orgasms, ejaculation, and the safe exchange of fluids.

Contraception as a whole is essential to women's health and the health of society, as is the ability to choose when or if to conceive. Whether that choice is based on personal reasons or based on medical circumstances that preclude the possibility of a healthy pregnancy, such as during illness, infection, or postpartum, contraception is what makes sexual and reproductive wellness possible. Contraception should be pain-free, safe, accessible, and tailored to each person's preferences and lifestyle.

The main methods of contraception today include barrier methods such as condoms, which not only prevent unwanted pregnancy but also protect against STIs. Hormonal birth control, and specifically the contraceptive pill, is by far the most commonly used contraceptive method, though it doesn't protect against STIs. Hormonal contraception may be prescribed for other reasons beside reproductive freedom: acne, migraines, and irregular cycles may lead health practitioners to hand out the pill.

Unfortunately, using the pill to "regulate" the menstrual cycle and hormonal cycle may result in a masking of symptoms that tend to return with a vengeance when hormonal contraception is discontinued—whether that is one year later or ten years later. In the past, medicinal herbs were used as contraceptive agents in the form of roots and seeds brewed as tea. These days, there are many different contraceptive methods to choose from. All contraceptive methods have pros and cons, benefits, risks, and potential side effects. The following section offers herbal recommendations for users of hormonal birth control, information on herbal contraceptives, and for when contraception fails, herbal support for pregnancy termination.

Hormonal Birth Control

Hormonal birth control is the most widely used form of contraception in the West today, and in the form of the contraceptive pill, it is convenient and easy to use. However, it is known to increase the risk of breast, cervical, and liver cancers. Other health risks associated with the pill include blood clot formation, stroke, heart disease, depression, weight gain, metabolic syndrome, and hormonal imbalance. Another unfortunate side effect of the pill, ironically, is a lower libido. This has led some health practitioners to quip: "The pill: it works; you won't risk getting pregnant because you'll never want to have sex again!"

What happens in the body as a result of prolonged exposure to hormonal birth control is a suppression of the menstrual cycle, which consists of ovulation, menstruation, and the hormonal flow that governs menses. Long-term use of hormonal contraceptives affects endocrine function, burdens the liver and other elimination pathways, and alters the flora populating the gut microbiome.

People with menstrual cycles who are sexually active and who wish to rely on hormonal contraception will find great support and relief from herbs to assist with renewed wellness and sexual and reproductive freedom. You can pair herbs with your current contraception method to relieve some of the associated health risks. Choice herbs for this purpose include lymphatics, nervines, cardiotonics, liver tonics, adaptogens, and nutritives.

Lymphatic herbs support hormonal balance by optimizing the function of elimination pathways. Optimal function of elimination pathways is essential for the clearance of excess hormones that may accumulate as a result of hormonal birth control use. The lymphatic system is no less essential than the blood circulatory system for human health and well-being and the cleansing of toxins from the body. Take the lymphatic tonic herbs calendula or cleavers or both daily, preferably in the form of infusions or herbal baths.

Nervine herbs support a healthy mood and nervous system. The use of hormonal birth control is associated with possible mood disorders, depression,[21] anxiety, and cancer of the central nervous system. Nervines replenish the nervous system and relax physical as well as mental and emotional strain. Herbal nervines include milky oats, valerian root, and passionflower. As a trophorestorative nervine, milky oats heal the myelin sheath and rebuild nerve tissue. They are often taken in the form of herbal tinctures.

Note that the popular antidepressant and nervine herb St. John's wort may interfere with birth control.[22] St. John's wort is an herbal cytochrome P450 inducer and is associated with increased metabolism of norethindrone and ethinyl estradiol, breakthrough bleeding, follicle growth, and ovulation.[23] In other words, it may interfere with contraceptive effectiveness and make it less effective.

Cardiotonic herbs keep the heart healthy. Hormonal birth control, and especially the pill, is linked with increased risk of heart disease, blood clots, and stroke. Cardiotonic herbs and heart tonics provide essential nourishment for cardiovascular health. Milky oats, hawthorn, and *Ginkgo biloba* are superior remedies to mitigate risk and support heart health and circulation. Flavonoids in *Ginkgo biloba* reduce capillary permeability and fragility, while also serving as free-radical scavengers.[24] Terpenes (in this case, ginkgolides) inhibit platelet-activating factor, lower vascular resistance, and enhance circulatory flow. *Ginkgo biloba* can be taken in capsule form.

Liver tonic herbs support liver health and detoxification. Hormonal contraception may tax the liver and overburden detoxification pathways.[25] A healthy liver and optimal hepatic function are necessary for the effective elimination of synthetic hormones from the body. Medicinal herbs for liver health include milk thistle, dandelion root, and turmeric. Enjoy these in tinctures or capsules. Turmeric can be made into delicious golden milk, a warm plant-based drink that's heartwarming and liver-healing at the same time.

Adaptogen herbs are superior endocrine regulators and hormonal balancers. They make ideal herbal allies for those who use hormonal birth control over long periods. Adaptogenic herbs and mushrooms such as holy basil (tulsi), reishi mushroom, and ashwagandha root regulate the HPA axis along with the ovary-adrenal-thyroid (OAT) axis. Enjoy holy basil in the form of daily infusions paired with nutritive and nervine herbs. Reishi and ashwagandha can be enjoyed in powder form, added to elixirs and smoothies.

Nutritive herbs deeply nourish your whole body and restore vitality and strength. The pill depletes specific vitamins and nutrients. Vitamin C, vitamin D, B vitamins, selenium, magnesium, and zinc are among the main nutrients that should be replenished with the help of medicinal herbs and nutritive tonics like nettle, oat straw, alfalfa, and dandelion leaf. Herbal tea brewed with nutritive herbs supplies the body with a wealth of highly bioavailable nutrients and helps reverse vitamin and mineral deficiency.

Herbal Post-Pill Cleansing

For those who are ready to forgo hormonal birth control, whether it is for medical or personal reasons, because their relationship ended, they want to practice celibacy, desire to try other contraceptive methods such as cycle charting and natural family planning, or are looking to have a baby, a period of post-pill cleansing is essential for bouncing back to optimal sexual and reproductive health.

Intentional post-pill cleansing nourishes and supports the body in finding its way back to hormonal balance and regular cycles. This is especially important for those who want to make a baby right away. A period of three to six months (and in some cases up to twelve months) of post-pill cleansing before conceiving can make a world of difference in the ease of conception and the experience of a healthy pregnancy, birth, and postpartum. But no matter whether or not baby-making is in the plans, post-pill cleansing with medicinal herbs brings the body back to balance by cleansing and restoring hormonal and sexual wellness.

Liver tonics support detoxification and clear out excess hormones. Liver tonic herbs include turmeric, milk thistle, and schisandra.

Nutritive tonics fill nutritional gaps and provide essential nutrients depleted by the pill. Nutritive tonic herbs include nettle, oat straw, red clover, and red raspberry leaf.

Uterine tonics tone the reproductive organs and nourish the uterus. Uterine tonic herbs include red raspberry leaf, lady's mantle, motherwort, and cramp bark.

Hormone balancers support a healthy hormonal cycle for menstrual wellness and fertility. Hormone balancing herbs include maca, vitex, milk thistle, and schisandra.

For a full protocol, follow all the recommendations included in the previous section, "Hormonal Birth Control," for current users of hormonal contraceptives.

Herbal Contraception

As more and more people become wary of using hormonal birth control, interest in herbal contraception is booming. Many women feel that they weren't appropriately warned by their doctors about the possible dangers and risks associated with hormonal contraceptives, and they are now looking for alternatives in the herb world. Along with a lack of trust in pharmaceuticals, there's also a lack of access to safe and welcoming sexual and reproductive health care for many women and people with female reproductive organs. All of this makes herbs and herbal contraception look like the haven at the end of the road. But are herbal contraceptives effective, and are they safe? It depends on whom you ask. I've dabbled in herbal contraception for a few years. Today, after ten years of herbal practice, my approach as a practitioner is to discourage the use of herbs as an ongoing contraceptive method.

Medicinal herbs make wonderful allies for sexual and reproductive wellness. They support optimal fertility and balanced hormones and cycles. But they're not the best option as a regular and ongoing method of contraception, for a few reasons. Using plants regularly to prevent conception means using plants to interrupt ovulation, to alter naturally occurring progesterone following ovulation (and to prevent implantation of a fertilized egg), or to otherwise disrupt important and finely tuned processes guided by the natural wisdom of the body. Even though there have been few, if any, modern reports of serious harm from responsible and educated herbal contraception, I'm not an advocate of using herbs to disrupt important and complex bodily processes. When my clients come to me asking for herbal contraception advice, I steer them toward cycle charting and body literacy instead.

Standard sex education has people believe that women are fertile all the time. The contraceptive pill, which is taken daily, reinforces this false notion. As a result, my clients think that in order to be effective, herbal contraception has to be taken daily as well. But women are only fertile for a handful of days each month. In order to be safe and effective, herbal contraception should be used only occasionally during this short fertile window.

In a cycle-aware, body-literate dreamland sex world of empowered fertility and conscious contraception, here is what would happen. Unprotected intercourse with penetration and ejaculation would take place during the infertile window (which usually means the luteal phase, during menstruation, and the beginning of the follicular phase—but every woman is different, so cycle-chart to be sure). During the fertile window (ovulation day plus the five to seven days prior), you would abstain from the type of sex that involves ejaculation inside the vagina or enjoy other yummy pleasures instead. Dildos, fingers, tongue—you name it, there's lots of options. If you really want penetrative sex during your fertile window, you would then use a nonhormonal barrier method like condoms.

What I recommend is only to use herbs as contraception in emergency cases, or as a backup when you slip from your responsible plan, or when the condom breaks. For folks with no access to pharmaceutical emergency birth control options like the morning-after pill, contraceptive herbs are useful to have on hand as an alternative. The approach I take with my clients is simple. Once they've become acquainted with and informed about their cycles and fertility, I may recommend small amounts of one herb to prevent implantation for emergency purposes: Queen Anne's lace. But with a few caveats.

Though little is known about herbal contraception today, medicinal herbs have been used for contraception and family planning for thousands of years. A huge loss of herbal knowledge occurred in the Middle Ages as a result of the witch hunts. Information regarding birth control was orally transmitted from woman to woman, and as a consequence of the persecution of "witches," who many believe were often female midwives, herbalists, and healers, much of this information was lost. But herbs continue to live on. Over 130 herbs have been identified by modern research as having antifertility properties. Medicinal plants affect fertility in distinct ways. Herbs may alter ovarian function, uterine function, and hormone production. They may inhibit hormonal action, implantation, and sperm production. Some herbs prevent fertilization by generating a protective layer around an egg. Antifertility plants prevent fertilization, antiovulatory plants inhibit ovulation, anti-implantation plants block implantation, and abortifacient plants cause abortion.

Queen Anne's lace, also called wild carrot *(Daucus carota),* is probably the best-known and most popular herb today when it comes to herbal contraception. I know many herb gals and friends who have relied on this herb for some years and with satisfaction. However, many folks have faced unwanted or unplanned pregnancies as a result of wild carrot use. There are a few kids in my social circle that we lovingly call "wild carrot babies." Wild carrot will have different outcomes based on when in the ovarian cycle it is consumed.

Queen Anne's lace is a biennial herb in the Apiaceae family. It has been known as a contraceptive herb with abortifacient and antifertility properties throughout history, and it is believed that wild carrot has been used in this way for over two thousand years. Modern North American herbalists suggest that oral administration of the seeds causes the endometrium to become inhospitable for a fertilized embryo to implant. The recommended protocol for using wild carrot seeds as contraception is to chew one teaspoon of seeds once a day during the ovulation period, or immediately after unprotected sex involving vaginal penetration and ejaculation during the fertile period of the menstrual cycle.

The fertility-enhancing properties of wild carrot are lesser known but potent, and like its antifertility properties, have to do with the phases of the menstrual cycle. Some women observe increased cervical secretions and vaginal lubrication when using wild carrot in the follicular phase leading up to ovulation. Wild carrot supports healthy estrogen levels in this phase of the cycle, which enhances wetness and libido and provides a receptive space for sperm and for conception to occur. Wild carrot also has gentle cleansing and detoxing properties that enhance health and fertility.

During the second phase of the menstrual cycle, known as the luteal phase, wild carrot seeds renew and refresh the womb by encouraging the shedding of old stagnant blood. In doing so, wild carrot may help promote conception and act as a fertility enhancer by preparing a fertile ground for a healthy embryo to be implanted during the following fertile period. But during or right after ovulation, wild carrot seeds can prevent eggs from implanting by encouraging the shedding of the uterine lining. In other words, wild carrot is pro-fertility during the follicular and luteal phases of the menstrual cycle. But during ovulation, it prevents implantation.

In this way, wild carrot may be used as both a pro-fertility and an anti-fertility agent. For enhancing fertility and the chances of conception, take the tinctured seed extract (15–30 drops) or chew 1 teaspoon of the seeds before ovulation. To prevent conception, take the same preparation during or right after ovulation and following unprotected intercourse. There are no clinical trials to draw data from when it comes to wild carrot seed and contraceptive purposes, but American herbalist Robin Bennett conducted an experiment in which twelve women from New York City used 1 teaspoon of Queen Anne's lace seeds for contraception for a duration of twelve months.[26] Her experiment concluded that the seeds were a very good method of contraception for those women who were willing to pay close attention to their cycles.

If you are interested in using wild carrot seeds, you will have to harvest them yourself in the late summer or autumn after the seeds have matured. Most herb stores do not carry them, though they are available through a couple of mail-order herb companies. Women with a history of kidney stones or gallstones should consult with an herbalist before using Queen

Anne's lace seeds. A standard dosage of 1 teaspoon of Queen Anne's lace seeds chewed daily during ovulation and continued for up to one week has worked effectively to prevent unwanted pregnancies for women of average height and build. If you are above average height or build, you might find the seeds more effective if you slightly raise the dosage.

Herbal Support for Pregnancy Endings, Miscarriages, and Abortion

Even the best contraceptive methods fail sometimes. No matter the reason why unwanted pregnancy happened, and why one may choose to end the pregnancy, herbs can be of great help and support both in a physiological and psychoemotional way. Unfortunately, even much wanted and anticipated pregnancies may also end in pregnancy loss. Abortion and miscarriage can cause physical, mental, and emotional stress and pain. Health concerns at this time include blood loss, low iron stores, fatigue, cramping and pain, stress, anxiety, PTSD, and hormonal swings. Herbs of special interest for the period following a pregnancy ending are nervine herbs, nutritives, adaptogens, antidepressant herbs, uterine tonics, and hormone balancers. Herbal care consists of calming the nervous system, providing the body with nutrients, and using herbs to support the reproductive organs.

A Note About Herbal Abortions, and Why They Should Be Avoided

There are reasons to believe that women have practiced abortions with various methods throughout time and history, and that this was widely accepted and respected as a part of women's health and agency as well as for the health and survival of families and communities. Emmenagogue herbs (herbs that help bring on menses) have been used to abort in previous times, as well as today in parts of the world where safe medical abortion is not available. But herbal abortions are potentially dangerous and should not be viewed as an alternative to accessible health care.

In recent years, as access to abortion and contraceptive services has come under attack by regressive agendas, many women have

resorted to herbalism as a way to provide reproductive wellness
for themselves and others. While sovereignty and autonomy are
essential to health, more must be done to fight for access to safe
and welcoming health care services for all. Restricting or denying
abortion access disproportionately impacts women, LGBTQ folks,
migrants, youth, poor folks, people living with disabilities, tired and
overworked single moms, and people of color. For post-abortion
care, however, medicinal herbs do have a lot to offer for recovery
and wellness.[27]

Nervine herbs provide soothing relief for mood balance and a tired nervous system. Hormonal changes may be strong in the period following
the pregnancy ending. Feelings of relief, sadness, elation, or depression
are common. Following an abortion, women are at a higher risk of mental
health problems such as anxiety, depression, and suicide. Some women
experience post–traumatic stress disorder (PTSD) following a miscarriage
or abortion. Meanwhile, nearly one in five women experience depression
or anxiety following a miscarriage. Psychoemotional symptoms can persist
for one to three years[28] and impact quality of life, relationships, family life,
careers, and subsequent pregnancies.

Along with herbal antidepressants and stress-reducing adaptogens,
herbal nervines make a healing addition to post-pregnancy loss protocols.
Milky oats extract contains phytochemicals such as the triterpenoid saponins avenacins that improve mood and protect against stress. Use of milky
oats benefits cognitive function and modulates the physiological response
to a stressor such as pregnancy ending. Enjoy it as an infusion, best paired
with nettle and red raspberry leaf.

Nutritive herbs nourish the body and bolster recovery from a pregnancy ending. Herbs with wide nutrient profiles and high amounts of bioavailable vitamins and minerals counter low iron associated with bleeding,
provide nutrients essential to uterine health, and keep the nervous system
nourished with nutrients associated with stable moods.

Nettle and yellow dock provide important sources of calcium, magnesium, iron, and vitamin C that prevent against anemia and fatigue. Milky

oats are rich in calcium, magnesium, and tryptophan, a precursor to the neurotransmitter serotonin (the "happy" hormone). Red raspberry leaf acts as an herbal nutritive and a uterine tonic. Nutritive herbs deliver the most benefit when they are enjoyed in the form of daily nourishing infusions.

Adaptogen herbs bring balance and equilibrium following a hormonally charged event. The impact of stress and high cortisol levels that may follow pregnancy loss make adaptogen herbs potential allies in the process. According to clinical herbalist Lisa Weiss,[29] specific adaptogens useful post-abortion include ashwagandha and shatavari.

Ashwagandha is an adaptogen as well as an immune stimulant, a calming nervine, and an antispasmodic useful for relieving cramping and pain, and it contains iron necessary for replenishing nutrition stores. As an adaptogen, ashwagandha acts as a mood stabilizer in clinical anxiety and depression. Ashwagandha and shatavari can be used in powder form and added to delicious plant-based elixirs, blended with nut milk and honey.

Antidepressant herbs may be useful following a pregnancy ending in miscarriage or abortion. From a hormonal perspective, the dip in estrogen and progesterone that characterizes pregnancy ending may cause depressive symptoms and low mood. Some women also experience pregnancy loss as a traumatic event, resulting in PTSD.

Symptoms of PTSD and depression include repetitive looping thoughts, excessive guilt, insomnia or oversleeping, hypervigilance, irritability, difficulty concentrating or focusing, reduced ability to make decisions, crying and weepiness, isolation, and suicidality. Herbal antidepressants include St. John's wort, mugwort, rosemary, lemon balm, passionflower, and damiana. Multiple clinical trials demonstrate the use of St. John's wort as an antidepressant. Mugwort acts as a mild nervine and antidepressant herb. Nervine herbs make pleasurable tinctures and can be taken daily, mixed with water or juice.

Uterine tonic herbs tone the uterus and reproductive organs. Heavy bleeding following miscarriage or abortion may warrant emergency care. However, if the bleeding is stable, uterine astringents can act as antihemorrhagic agents on the uterus. With or without bleeding, uterine tonics are recommended to strengthen the reproductive system.

Motherwort offers uterine support in the event of prolonged bleeding after a medical abortion. Red raspberry leaf, a prime uterine tonic and nutritive tonic herb, improves nutrition and circulation to the uterus and acts as an astringent tonic to relieve bleeding and pain. If painful cramps and spasms cause discomfort, uterine antispasmodics like valerian, cramp bark, wild yam, and ginger can be taken as needed in tincture form for fast and effective relief.

Hormone-balancing herbs mediate and regulate hormonal shifts. For most women, hormone levels return to normal pre-pregnancy levels within the first menstrual cycle post-abortion, and within one to nine weeks following a miscarriage. Still, hormone balancing herbs bring relief and assist the return back to reproductive wellness and balanced cycles following a pregnancy ending.

Vitex restores hormone balance, normalizes reproductive function, and reduces inflammation of the endometrium. Clinical herbalist Lisa Weiss points out that if sex hormones are having trouble returning to normal, liver function should be examined. In any case, liver herbs do have a positive influence on hormone balance: schisandra, milk thistle, and dandelion may be added to the herbal protocol for this liver-healing purpose. Use these liver herbs in tincture form or in capsules.

Taking care of your body, heart, and psyche at this time is essential. Reach out if you need help, and let herbs be your allies through the process. In this way, you'll be joining a long and ancient lineage of women and mothers who have walked this path alongside you since time immemorial.

Endometriosis

Endometriosis is a chronic, estrogen-dependent disorder affecting women in which endometrial tissue (the endometrium) grows abnormally and adheres outside the uterus.[30] The most common site for wayward endometrium is the ovaries, but lesions also occur on the fallopian tubes, pelvic ligaments, and the outside of the uterus, bowel, and bladder. Called "endo" for short, it is one of the most common gynecological diseases and affects 10 to 20 percent of women of reproductive age. Because of the chronic, repetitive nature of the disorder, it can be considered a hormonal imbalance, an autoimmune disorder, and a disability.

The most common symptoms associated with endometriosis are chronic pelvic pain as well as insanely painful menstrual cramping, also called dysmenorrhea (but with endo, it's more like dysmenorrhea on steroids). Constipation and bloating, fatigue, lower-back pain and pain that radiates down the inner thighs, pain during sex, and urinary problems as well as pain while peeing are other symptoms associated with endometriosis. In some cases, inflammation and scarring from endometrial lesions may lead to infertility. As can be expected with a condition linked with such persistent pain and no known cure, endometriosis causes possible mood swings, depression, and anxiety in those who live with the disease. Endometriosis is considered a disabling condition that may significantly compromise social relationships, sexuality, and mental health.[31]

What Causes Endometriosis?

Many factors are possible causes for endometriosis. In recent years there has been growing concern that endometriosis is linked with endocrine disruptors and other chemicals present in the environment.[32] Toxic exposure to artificial chemicals such as dioxins and dioxin-like compounds increases the burden on the body. This in turn leads to inflammation and hormonal disruptions like those associated with endo.

There is no known cure for endometriosis, but alleviating symptoms is possible. Conventional treatment for the disease includes the continued use of pain medications for symptom management and the removal of endometrial tissue via the surgical procedure known as a laparoscopy. As a last resort, a total hysterectomy may be performed. This involves the removal of the uterus via surgery and may also involve removal of the cervix, ovaries, fallopian tubes, and other surrounding structures, which ends a woman's chances of ever becoming pregnant and carrying a baby.

Conventional treatment for endometriosis carries numerous health risks and potential for trauma for women,[33] who routinely endure many misdiagnoses and invasive procedures on their journey to a pain-free, endo-free life.

For women living with endometriosis, whether its symptoms are light or severe, herbal remedies can help. Herbs relieve symptoms and support the body in finding equilibrium on both a physical and emotional level. Several studies observing the effects of traditional Chinese herbal remedies on endometriosis have shown highly beneficial results.[34] Herbs relieve dysmenorrhea, shrink ectopic lesions, and promote fertility. The remedies tested include dong quai, ginseng, skullcap, and ginger.

The main goals of herbal support with endometriosis are to manage pain, reduce inflammation, enhance detoxification pathways, support liver health, balance hormones, tone and support the health of the reproductive organs, and soothe emotional pain, stress, and worry. Medicinal herbs useful in the context of endometriosis support include pain-relieving, anti-inflammatory, and antioxidant herbs; hepatics; hormone-balancing herbs; uterine tonics; antidepressant herbs; and nervines.[35]

Turmeric is an excellent herbal remedy for endometriosis. The high antioxidant, anti-inflammatory capacity of turmeric paired with its liver-supporting ability makes it a supreme ally for living with endometriosis and relieving its symptoms. One of the main active compounds of turmeric, curcumin, plays a major role in the control of inflammation, cell proliferation, and angiogenesis in both animal and human studies.[36] As an antiangiogenic compound, curcumin effectively stops endometrial lesions from growing and stops endometriosis from spreading.[37]

Studies show that both curcumin as well as herbal formulas containing turmeric significantly alleviate and improve the symptoms of endo patients.[38] Turmeric lowers inflammation and reverses oxidative stress and free-radical damage. As a liver herb, it cleanses the liver pathways and enhances the clearing of excess estrogen from the body. Finally, turmeric helps with pain management. It is especially powerful for pain relief when it is combined with ginger. The healing herb combo works wonders without the dangerous side effects associated with the prescription meds commonly used with endo. For best results, take turmeric and ginger in capsule form.

Milk thistle supports the health of people living with endometriosis. The seed of milk thistle acts as a potent hepatic tonic. Silymarin and its active constituent, silybin, are antioxidants found in milk thistle that stabilize mast cells in the liver, increase protein production in liver cells, and protect the liver against damage. The liver is responsible for clearing out toxins from the body, including excess hormones like estrogen. Because endometrial lesions depend on estrogen for development and growth, liver tonic herbs like milk thistle become valuable remedies for people with endo. Use milk thistle in tincture form or in capsules.

Supporting the liver in the context of endo serves a two-fold purpose: first, better liver health keeps estrogen levels in check, which stops endo growth and spread. Second, endo sufferers commonly need pain medication in order to keep pain down to manageable levels. Consumption of pain medication makes liver dysfunction a major concern. There is strong potential for the pain of endometriosis to require more pain medication, which further burdens the liver, causing a worsening in endometriosis symptoms, thus requiring more pain meds. But milk thistle and silymarin can put a stop to this dangerous loop. Anti-inflammatory and liver supportive, silymarin has been found by science to be not only effective in the management of endo symptoms but a therapeutic agent for the treatment of endometriosis as well.[39]

Medicinal mushrooms address the autoimmune roots of endometriosis. Isolated metabolites from medicinal mushrooms modulate immune responses and lower inflammation.[40] Medicinal mushrooms useful in the context of endometriosis include reishi, turkey tail, shiitake, cordyceps, and lion's mane. As immune-modulating adaptogens, medicinal mushrooms maintain the body in a state of harmony and balance. They provide important antioxidants to reverse the oxidative stress and free-radical damage that worsen endometriosis symptoms. Enjoy medicinal mushrooms in the form of powder, tincture, or capsule.

Reishi and turkey tail are potent liver-supporting remedies that cleanse the liver and free the body of toxins and excess hormones. Medicinal mushrooms enhance cognitive function and boost energy levels in both a physical and a mental way. As such, they make an ideal companion for the brain fog and fatigue associated with endo and its symptoms. People living with endometriosis find that adding medicinal mushrooms to their wellness regimen alleviates symptoms of endo while increasing quality of life and the ability to enjoy their health journey from a more resourced place.

Pain-relieving herbs and herbal painkillers relieve pain in the pelvis and abdomen. They include black cohosh, ginger, turmeric, chamomile, and dong quai.

Antispasmodic herbs relieve cramps, soothe sharp and dull pain, and relieve pain in the lower back and thighs. They include wild yam, black haw, black cohosh, chamomile, and ginger. These herbs are also useful as anti-inflammatory herbs for pain in the uterus, intestines, bowel, and urinary system.

Sedative herbs support deep rest and sleep and provide relief from pain. They include valerian, hops, and California poppy. In small doses, they can be calming and pain-relieving. In larger doses, they may put you to sleep.

Nervines and antidepressant herbs assist with mood balance and relieve stress, anxiety, and tension. They include milky oats, passionflower, St. John's wort, and damiana.

Immune balancing herbs for immunological conditions coexisting with endometriosis include echinacea, astragalus, ashwagandha, ginseng, rhodiola, reishi, and cordyceps.

Immuno-supportive and anti-inflammatory adaptogen herbs for hyperimmunity and autoimmune disorders with endometriosis include licorice, ashwagandha, and American ginseng.

Lymphatic tonic herbs for enhanced lymph flow and circulation include calendula, echinacea, cleavers, and poke root (*Phytolacca*).

Erectile Dysfunction

The experience of erectile dysfunction is common for men. It can be linked to several different conditions of reproductive health and sexual function. Adult men of any age can be affected by it, though the likelihood of erectile dysfunction increases with age and may affect more than half of all men over age fifty. It's interesting to note that while older men have a higher rate of erectile dysfunction overall, younger men may experience more severe cases of it.[41]

Erectile dysfunction is defined as the inability to maintain an erection sufficient for sexual intercourse. As such, it has the potential to severely affect a man's sensual, embodied enjoyment of sexual activity that includes penetration, thrusting, and ejaculation. Male sexual function is divided into three main components: libido and desire for sexual activity, ability to get and keep a strong erection, and finally, orgasm and ejaculation.

> Previously known as "impotence," the term has now been updated to reflect that the experience of erectile dysfunction doesn't define a man, as in being an "impotent man." Rather, the condition carries symptoms such as soft erections and may be treated with various protocols. This condition does not define a man and his ability to be sexually healthy.

The achievement of an erection is a complex process involving the brain, hormones, nerves, muscles, and blood flow. If an instrument misses the tempo through the process of this finely tuned orchestra, the result may be erectile dysfunction. Conventional treatment for erectile dysfunction includes the go-to "blue pill," PDE5 inhibitors like Viagra and Cialis.

PDE5 is an enzyme in the walls of blood vessels. By inhibiting this enzyme, the blood vessels relax and blood flow is increased. This type of medication will work to relieve the symptoms of erectile dysfunction for many men, enabling them to return to a sexual potency that might vastly increase quality of life and relational satisfaction. But up to 40 percent of men don't experience benefits from the blue pill at all. That's because its efficacy or lack thereof depends on the root cause of erectile dysfunction.

PDE5 inhibitors dilate blood vessels and increase blood flow to the penis. If erectile dysfunction is caused by poor blood flow to the penis, the medication works wonders. But if erectile dysfunction stems from different causes, which for many men it does, these medications will have zero benefit.

Possible causes and risk factors for erectile dysfunction include heart disease, coronary artery disease, high blood pressure, metabolic syndrome, diabetes, obesity, depression, low testosterone levels, kidney disease, and prostate cancer. Psychological or emotional causes for erectile dysfunction include sexual performance anxiety, self-consciousness around a new sexual partner, confusion with sexual identity or gender attraction, or a generalized state of depression or burnout that extinguishes the flames of Eros. Finally, there are strong indications that racism and oppression contribute to the prevalence of erectile dysfunction as well.

Though few studies have observed the racial disparity in the prevalence of erectile dysfunction, the two main risk factors for erectile dysfunction—cardiovascular disease and diabetes—disproportionately affect Black people, indigenous people, and people of color (BIPOC). Black adults and Hispanics score higher than White and Asian folks on risk factors associated with heart disease, such as hypertension and obesity.[42] Meanwhile, a study on the impact of type 2 diabetes mellitus found that 16 percent of indigenous men were affected, compared with 6.2 percent of nonindigenous men.[43] Unemployment and low income may also negatively affect a man's chance of remission post–erectile dysfunction, which means that unemployed and low-income men may react more poorly to conventional treatment.[44]

There are many reasons to look to medicinal herbs as a valued support for erectile dysfunction. Healing herbs address a wealth of symptoms and risk factors related to erectile dysfunction, from heart health to stress, diabetes, depression, and low libido. Herbs can be taken safely for long periods and can treat the root cause of erectile dysfunction. In this way, herbs differ from medications like Viagra and other PDE5 inhibitors, which carry numerous side effects and may lose efficacy over long periods of use. PDE5 inhibitors don't address the root causes of erectile dysfunction, but herbs do.

For men of all ages, virility-boosting herbs can be enjoyed recreationally and to reverse erectile dysfunction, make a strong erection even stronger, increase lasting power, crank up the intensity of orgasm, and shorten refractory time post-ejaculation. Men and their sexual partners have enjoyed healing herbs in this way for thousands of years. Herbs are celebrated for their effect on erections, arousal, orgasm, and sexual ability in the ancient medicine systems of Traditional Chinese Medicine and Ayurveda, with choice herbs like ginseng used to tone the entire male sexual and reproductive system. Tonic herbs for sexual health blend together the therapeutic, the curative, and the pleasurable. Men find that the addition of healing herbs to their holistic sexual health tool kit enables them to support their health in both physiological, emotional, mental, relational, and physical ways.

When dealing with erectile dysfunction, it is essential to work with your health providers to establish the most probable cause for the condition. Based on the cause at play, either one or several of the following herbal protocols for erectile dysfunction may be indicated. As far as individual herbs go, ginseng and maca are significant for men looking to increase sexual stamina and prevent erectile dysfunction while supporting overall health.

Ginseng is a stimulating adaptogen and a superior herbal remedy for erectile dysfunction. Many types of ginseng share similar properties. *Panax ginseng* is the Asian ginseng most commonly used in the context of erectile dysfunction and in the promotion of healthy erections. The benefits of ginseng root on erectile function are often attributed to the ginsenosides present in the plant. The active plant constituents in ginseng are ginsenosides, a class of steroid glycosides and triterpene saponins.[45] They promote nitric oxide release, trigger erection, and relax smooth muscle, allowing for more blood flow and an enlarged penis.

Ginseng improves cardiovascular function and decreases risk factors associated with erectile dysfunction, such as hypertension, hyperglycemia, and hyperlipidemia. Ginseng is a natural sexual tonic that boosts sexual stamina and arousal, lifts energy levels, and reverses fatigue. *Panax ginseng* is recommended for use in older men and elders. For young men, other types of ginseng are preferred, such as Siberian ginseng, also called eleuthero *(Eleutherococcus senticosus),* which possesses more balanced adaptogenic properties and is less stimulating. Enjoy ginseng as a tincture or in capsule form.

Wild American ginseng *(Panax quinquefolius)* should not be harvested, used, or consumed, as it is listed as an endangered plant. However, it can be cultivated sustainably and is a popular crop within nontimber forest products initiatives around North America.

Maca is a nutrient-rich root vegetable from the Peruvian Andes and a popular sexual tonic. The potential active constituents in maca include macaridine, macamides, macaene, glucosinolates, maca alkaloid, and maca nutrients.[46] My experience suggests that maca may be effective for folks with erectile dysfunction after twelve weeks of treatment with maca root extract. Dosage varies from 1.5 grams of powder per day to 3 grams of powder per day. Maca is an adaptogen and hormone-balancing herb with many other benefits to overall health. It is also used for physical endurance, energy, and stamina, making maca an ideal companion to sexual vitality for men.

Maca is highly tolerable with little to no health risks or side effects, has a great safety profile, and possesses low risk to no risk of interactions with medication. As such, it makes a smart and reliable option for men looking for natural ways to address erectile dysfunction. No matter the cause of erectile dysfunction, maca may provide benefits and symptom relief. In fact, maca root is investigated in human clinical trials as an adjuvant therapy to treat antidepressant-related sexual dysfunction.[47] Men who consume maca regularly report better sleep, more energy, less stress, and better sexual function overall. Enjoy maca in the form of powder added to smoothies, capsules, or liquid extract.

How safe is maca? The only negative effect of maca I could find in the scientific literature involved a thirty-year-old man who showed up at a military hospital after consuming 300 milliliters of maca tincture in 50 percent alcohol.[48] He suffered jaundice as a result, and his clinical condition and liver function soon recovered from the initial hit—though his liver remained impacted for some time. No one in their right mind would consume such an enormous amount of maca tincture, however. The recommended daily dosage for maca is 1 milliliter three times daily. So this man consumed one hundred times more than the recommended daily dose of maca extract, and the 300 milliliters of strong alcohol probably didn't help either. My estimate is this equaled about seven shots of hard liquor—yikes! In any case, this story illustrates just how safe maca really is—imagine taking a hundred times the dose of anything and coming out fine.

Erectile dysfunction and cardiovascular disorders often go hand in hand. Herbs that support both systems at once include the circulatory stimulants *Ginkgo biloba* and rosemary, along with the cardiotonics milky oats and hawthorn for heart health.

A healthy prostate also supports a healthy sexual function in men. Prostate conditions like benign prostate hyperplasia (BPH) and prostate cancer treatment are known to affect erectile function—and vice versa. For example, men with erectile dysfunction are 1.33 to 6.24 times more likely to experience BPH than men without erectile dysfunction.[49] Medicinal herbs with a beneficial impact on prostate health and erectile dysfunction include saw palmetto and nettle root.

Finally, stress, anxiety, and tension contribute to erectile dysfunction. Deeply restorative and rejuvenating adaptogen herbs to support the nervous system include ashwagandha root and reishi mushroom. Adaptogens increase resistance to stress, both from physical, mental, environmental, and emotional stressors. Episodes of depression and other mood disorders affect men's ability to enjoy sexual intimacy and have been correlated with erectile dysfunction.

At the same time, the use of antidepressants causes erectile dysfunction in some men. Medicinal herbs with an affinity for erectile dysfunction and depression include the antidepressant herb damiana along with circulatory stimulant and tonic herb *Ginkgo biloba*. In an open trial, *Ginkgo biloba* was found to be 76 percent effective in treating antidepressant-induced sexual dysfunction predominantly caused by selective serotonin reuptake inhibitors (SSRIs) in men.[50]

Fertility

As part of my herbal practice, I recommend that everyone commits to a fertility promoting protocol with medicinal herbs. Herbal protocols that support fertility are also supporting overall sexual and reproductive health and function. Most of the adaptogenic hormone-balancing aphrodisiacs I recommend for fertility also happen to be delightful health enhancers with impacts reaching far beyond conception and baby-making and rippling through better immune health and hormonal balance. The topics addressed in this section include an overview of the female and male reproductive systems as they relate to fertility. Medicinal herbs most useful for enhancing fertility are discussed, followed by herbal protocols well suited in conjunction with fertility treatments.

Infertility

Infertility is defined as the lack of conception after twelve consecutive months of attempting to become pregnant. Ten to fifteen percent of couples experience infertility, and this number is growing fast. Various factors affect a couple's ability to conceive. About one-third of infertility cases are caused by female factors while another third are caused by male factors. The remaining third of infertility cases are caused by a combination of female and male factors or by unexplained factors. After all, even though conception seems at first glance like a pretty straightforward process, many conditions must be met in order for pregnancy to happen. A woman must ovulate, sperm must be present, regular intercourse must occur during the window of fertility, and the fallopian tubes and uterus must be up to the task.

The most common female factors that decrease fertility include disorders with ovulation such as PCOS, damaged fallopian tubes, endometriosis, and problems with the uterus or cervix. Male factors that influence fertility include physical conditions of the reproductive system and semen count and quality. Herbs are used as a treatment for infertility in a variety of ways. Herbs regulate the menstrual cycle, which in turn increases regularity of ovulation. Herbs tone the reproductive organs, increase libido, enhance lubrication and vaginal wetness, increase sperm count, and heighten sperm mobility.

Female Fertility

The female reproductive system is a combination of external structures, including the vaginal opening and clitoris, and internal reproductive organs, including the vagina, the uterus, ovaries, and fallopian tubes. During the reproductive years the female reproductive system undergoes a menstrual cycle, controlled by hormones within the body.

During a healthy menstrual cycle, the body prepares for a pregnancy (follicular phase), and if conception does not occur at the time of ovulation (ovulatory phase), the body releases the preparation for pregnancy as a menstrual period (luteal phase). The menstrual cycle is on average twenty-eight days long with ovulation occurring at day 14, but this can vary significantly from body to body. This information is often used in predicting which days to have intercourse for the purpose of conception.

Tracking the female menstrual cycle using the fertility awareness method (FAM) enhances a woman's ability to understand her cycle and accurately determine which days are the best for achieving or avoiding pregnancy. Healthy functioning of the female reproductive system is controlled by an assemblage of hormones operating in tandem. FSH and LH are released during the follicular phase, when the release of these two hormones causes the release of estrogen. When estrogen reaches a certain level, FSH is shut off.

Estrogen, produced by a dominant follicle in one ovary, surges during the ovulatory phase, causing the release of LH. At this point a mature egg is released from the follicle into the fallopian tube. The empty follicular structure becomes the corpus luteum in the luteal phase, where it releases estrogen and progesterone. Progesterone is responsible for preparing the uterus for successful implantation. If conception occurs, the egg will travel out of the fallopian tube and implant into the uterus. If conception does not occur, the egg and the lining of the uterus are shed during menstruation. If something goes awry through this process, infertility may arise.

Male Fertility

The male reproductive system consists of external and internal components as well. The external components include the penis, scrotum, and testicles. Internally, the male reproductive system includes the vas deferens, prostate, and urethra. This system is responsible for the production of sperm, semen, and sex hormones. The testicles (testes) are located within the scrotum and are responsible for the production of sex hormones and semen. Sperm produced by the testes reside within the epididymis until they reach maturation and travel into the vas deferens during sexual arousal. The vas deferens then transports the semen into the urethra for ejaculation.

Similar to the female reproductive system, the male system is under the control of hormones. The primary hormones involved in male reproductive function include FSH, LH, and testosterone. These hormones are released by the pituitary gland, located at the base of the brain. FSH is mainly responsible for the production of sperm, whereas LH contributes to the production of testosterone. Testosterone itself influences the development of secondary sex characteristics in the male body, like the distribution of hair and muscle mass.

Some of the main conditions that affect the male reproductive system include various cancers such as prostate or testicular cancers, enlarged prostate, prostatitis, infertility, and hormone imbalances like testosterone deficiency. Infertility may be influenced by lifestyle factors such as diet, exercise, and smoking, along with environmental exposure to toxins. Most often male infertility is linked to low sperm count and low sperm motility, meaning the sperm has trouble reaching the egg for the purpose of fertilization.

Fertility Herbs

Ashwagandha is an adaptogen herb, general tonic, nervous system tonic, and aphrodisiac. It is beneficial for testicular health and increased fertility via both stress reduction, higher sperm quality, and higher sperm count. Ashwagandha boosts fertility by helping to balance the hormones within the body.

Eleuthero is an adaptogen and tonic. It is also called Siberian ginseng and boosts endurance, stamina, and focus. Eleuthero increases sperm count and relieves erectile dysfunction while also supporting the health of the body as a whole.

Ginseng is a tonic herb with benefits for physiological and sexual function. Ginseng aids with erectile dysfunction (particularly in combination with ginkgo and rhodiola) and low sperm count. Ginseng increases male libido, penile rigidity, girth, and duration of erection.[51] Ginseng reduces abnormalities in sperm. It increases sperm count and motility as well as testosterone levels. Ginseng protects the testes from environmental pollutants by fighting free radicals and protecting the cell membrane.

Lady's mantle is a tonic to the female reproductive organs and balances menstrual flow either by bringing on a delayed period or decreasing menstrual flow, which improves fertility.

Maca is an adaptogen and potent nutritive. It is rich in vitamins and minerals. Maca provides energy and vitality and increases sperm production, sperm quality, and overall fertility. As a hormone balancer, maca leads to heightened libido and sexual desire.

Nettle is a reproductive system tonic and nutritive herb. Nettle root has a strong affinity for the prostate gland and reduces inflammation. Nettle leaf acts as a potent nutritive and regenerates the sexual and reproductive organs, increasing sperm count and seminal fluids. Nettle leaf is rich in trace minerals and amino acids to restore the enzymes and antioxidants necessary for protecting sperm cells.

Red raspberry leaf is a trusted best friend for women in their reproductive years. This plant is useful for those desiring pregnancy, since the fragrine component tones the uterus and all reproductive organs.

Saw palmetto is used for bladder disorders, lowered sex drive and libido, hormone imbalances, BPH, and prostate cancer.

Schisandra is an adaptogen and aphrodisiac. It is a liver trophorestorative that supports hormonal balance and reproductive health. Schisandra supports healthy fertility.

Shatavari is an Ayurvedic rejuvenating tonic herb. It is an adaptogen, aphrodisiac, reproductive tonic, and fertility builder. It balances hormones, with a beneficial action on the menstrual cycle and pelvic inflammatory diseases. It increases vaginal lubrication.

Vitex has progesterone-type activity within the body and improves menstrual regularity. Vitex should not be used in conjunction with the female contraceptive pill, fertility treatments, or hormone therapies. Where problems of infertility are linked to hormonal imbalance (as opposed to physical factors), vitex is used to bring balance to estrogen and progesterone release throughout the menstrual cycle. Remedying this imbalance leads to improved chances of conception.

Wild yam is a hormone regulator. It supports the estrogen-progesterone balance due to its diosgenin content, a precursor of steroid hormones. Wild yam regulates the menstrual cycle and supports fertility. As a liver tonic herb, wild yam helps the liver in synthesizing sex hormones with a beneficial impact on hormonal imbalances.

Fertility and Common Pollutants

Common harmful pollutants that affect fertility include bisphenol A (BPA), dioxins, heavy metals, and phthalates. BPA is an industrial plastic softener. It is one of the leading causes of occupational infertility. BPA acts as both an endocrine disruptor and a metabolic disruptor, which mimics the effect of estrogen in the body. Even in low doses, BPA affects the timing of puberty, reduces sperm count, and enlarges the prostate. It is linked to infertility[52] and may impair ovarian development and disrupt follicular and uterine morphology.

From an herbal perspective, ashwagandha root offers protection against BPA-induced oxidative stress and toxicity.[53] Reduce exposure to BPA as much as possible and take ashwagandha root daily in the form of tincture, capsules, or powder.

Dioxins and furans are bioaccumulative contaminants. They are mainly generated through the burning of petrochemicals like oil, plastic, and coal. These materials are very persistent in the environment and accumulate in the fat cells of animals and humans. Dioxins are of significant concern because of their accumulative nature. This process is known as biomagnification. Dioxins are carcinogenic, immunosuppressant, and potent endocrine disruptors. Studies show that infertile men have higher concentrations of these dioxins in their seminal fluid compared with fertile men.[54] Dioxin exposure is linked with pelvic pain and subfertility in women with endometriosis.[55]

Antioxidant herbs protect against the damages caused by dioxin exposure. Turmeric and chaga mushroom offer antioxidant protection from oxidative damage and toxicity induced by dioxin accumulation. Dong quai has been studied for its free-radical scavenging ability in the context of dioxin toxicity.[56] Herbal remedies effective against dioxin toxicity blend dandelion, licorice, and other herbs for enhanced detoxification and elimination of harmful substances from the body.[57]

Heavy metals enter the environment as waste products from mining and fossil-fuel extraction. Many agrochemicals, like fertilizers and pesticides, are derived from petrochemicals and contain heavy metal contaminants.[58] Lead, mercury, cadmium, arsenic, copper, aluminum, and lithium are some of the most common heavy metals affecting fertility today. Lead and cadmium especially have strong antifertility effects. They disrupt hormone balance, significantly lower semen quality, and cause genetic damage as they accumulate in the testicles.

From an herbal perspective, these heavy metals can be removed from the body through chelation. The blue-green alga chlorella, for instance, acts as a natural chelator of heavy metals, especially lead and mercury, due to its high chlorophyll content. For best results, take concentrated chlorella tablets. Chlorella and cilantro consumed as food detoxify neurotoxins like the heavy metal mercury as well as toxic chemicals like phthalates, plasticizers, and insecticides.[59] Medicinal herbs with strong chelation properties include *Ginkgo biloba,* milk thistle, and triphala.

Phthalates are widely used for waterproofing food and beverage containers and in the manufacturing of automobiles, medical equipment, and the ubiquitous plastics that litter the earth and waters around the world. Phthalates disrupt the hypothalamic-pituitary-gonadal (HPG) axis, which includes the ovaries in women and testes in men, by disrupting the binding of hormones to their receptor sites, serving as an antagonist.

Detoxifying herbs reduce the chemical burden of phthalate exposure. Milk thistle seed, a potent liver tonic, along with dandelion root are great allies for phthalates detox. Pharmacological studies show that dandelion extract has hepatoprotective effects against chemical agents, thanks to its antioxidant and anti-inflammatory activities.[60] The anti-inflammatory effects of dandelion, the prebiotic effects of its oligofructans, and its many other healing factors greatly improve liver function, enhance the elimination of the toxic burden, and reduce the allostatic load from chemical exposure. I like to make a composed tincture blend with milk thistle seed and dandelion root. I recommend taking this daily for a one-month period for this purpose. Repeat this seasonally as a regular cleanse.

Herbs and Fertility Treatments

Folks struggling with fertility may wonder what herbs they can safely take along with fertility treatment like medications and assisted reproductive technologies. It is probably wise to avoid hormonal herbs during fertility treatments, as potential interactions have not been appropriately measured through time.

The support of an experienced endocrinologist and a clinical herbalist together would be appropriate for making personalized recommendations when it comes to combining herbs with a potential for hormonal activity along with medical fertility treatment.

An interaction has been noted between vitex and in vitro fertilization (IVF), for example.[61] A thirty-two-year-old woman took vitex extract before and in the early follicular phase of her fourth cycle of unstimulated IVF treatment. Her reasoning was to use vitex to help promote ovarian function. In this cycle, she developed four follicles rather than the normal one, and her serum gonadotrophin and ovarian hormone measurements grew out of balance.

She stopped the vitex supplementation and soon experienced symptoms that suggested mild ovarian hyperstimulation syndrome in the luteal phase of her menstrual cycle. After discontinuing vitex, the two following cycles were normal, with one follicle developed. The three cycles previous to vitex supplementation were also normal. This suggests that hormonal herbs should be avoided during IVF treatment due to their unpredictable outcomes.

On the other hand, some randomized clinical trials show a positive link between Chinese herbs and IVF outcomes.[62] Another study has shown promise in combining herbal remedies along with clomiphene citrate (Clomid) in infertile women with PCOS.[63] An herbal blend with mint, ginger, and other medicinal herbs had a beneficial action on serum antioxidant levels as well as glycemic biomarkers of infertile polycystic ovary syndrome. The herbal blend also enhanced menstrual regulation and promoted a higher pregnancy rate. These positive correlations between herbs and pregnancy outcomes for fertility patients are worth exploring further.

One area where folks struggling with fertility and undergoing medical fertility treatment will strongly and safely benefit from herbs is in increasing quality of life and nourishing the emotional body. Folks experiencing infertility are at higher risk for emotional distress, depression, anxiety, low self-esteem, and general anguish that is infertility specific.

What's more, soothing and relieving emotional difficulties increases the success rates of fertility treatment.[64] Herbs with a strong affinity for the emotional realm, for soothing the nerves, and for helping relieve depression are welcomed in this protocol. Lemon balm, damiana, passionflower, and milky oats are potent healing herbs in the process of your fertility journey. They make every day gentler and kinder, and keep your heart wide open to the miracles of life, Eros, and creation.

Hemorrhoids

Hemorrhoids are swollen veins in the rectum that cause severe pain and discomfort and difficulty in passing bowel movements. Hemorrhoids affect folks of all ages and all genders. They are common during pregnancy, especially in the third trimester, because increased blood flow to the pelvic area as well as pressure from the enlarged uterus and growing baby can cause the veins that run through the anus to swell. Hemorrhoids also tend to affect the elderly because of age-related changes in the blood vessels along with potential sedentary behavior and constipation.

Hemorrhoids range in severity from grade 1 to grade 4, based on whether they are internal or prolapsed, and bleeding or not bleeding. A mild episode of hemorrhoids might consist of swollen tender veins in the rectum, while a severe episode might involve painful swollen veins poking outside the anus (prolapsed) that may rupture and bleed. Anal sex can make mild hemorrhoids worse, but gentle self-massage on the anal region has been considered by some sexual health practitioners to be healing and beneficial to recovery because it promotes healthy blood circulation and relaxes the muscular tension in the lower back and buttocks.

Herbal therapies offer great promise in the treatment of hemorrhoids, naturally. The protocol serves two purposes: first, to soothe pain and swelling in the anal area for symptom relief. The second goal is to address the root causes of hemorrhoids and help reverse the condition over long-term use of herbs by working with the venous system. The main herbs used in the context of hemorrhoids include anti-inflammatory and wound-healing plantain, comfrey, St. John's wort, calendula, red raspberry leaf, and circulatory tonics like gotu kola and horse chestnut.

To relieve the symptoms associated with hemorrhoids, an herbal oil or salve is applied locally for anti-inflammatory action and to relieve pain and itch. Use plantain, comfrey, St. John's wort, and calendula as an herbal base. Apply liberally as many times a day as needed. Use a blend of antibacterial herbs along with wound-healing and anti-inflammatory herbs for best results.

Plantain is a potent anti-inflammatory herb with strong effect to relieve itch, swelling, and pain. Comfrey is a wound healer to speed healing and fortify the affected tissues. St. John's wort is an antibacterial and anti-inflammatory herb to keep the affected area clean and relieve swelling. Calendula is a soothing and wound-healing antibacterial herb with a strong affinity with the anal mucosa.

Herbal sitz baths are used for fast healing and recovery from hemorrhoids. For those who experience chronic recurrences, sitz baths may be an ideal preventative measure to protect against hemorrhoids. Red raspberry leaf and other astringent herbs are ideal for this purpose. Red raspberry leaf is a beneficial astringent herb that tightens and tones loose, red, and inflamed tissue. This herb can be swapped out for blackberry leaf or yarrow for similar results in a sitz bath.

Witch hazel water is also highly indicated in the context of herbal soaks for healing hemorrhoids. Steep a strong herbal tea and strain into the bath, filling the tub halfway. Let the lower body and pelvic area soak in the tea for at least twenty minutes. Repeat up to four times per day until symptoms subside during acute episodes, or up to three or four times weekly as prevention.

Internal remedies, which are ingested, are used for venous health and tightening of the loose tissues associated with prolapsed and swollen hemorrhoids. Gotu kola and horse chestnut are the most significant. Internal remedies may be taken in the form of tincture or herbal capsules and for long periods. Gotu kola is used for venous insufficiency and to strengthen connective tissue. Horse chestnut is approved by the German Commission E for chronic venous insufficiency (CVI).

One double-blind placebo-controlled study on eighty patients suffering from acute symptomatic hemorrhoids demonstrated that aescin, one of the active compounds in horse chestnut, reduced hemorrhoid symptoms in 81 percent of the subjects, compared to 11 percent in the placebo group.[65] Bleeding was also reduced in the horse chestnut group (95 percent versus 62 percent) and so was swelling (87 percent versus 38 percent). The dosage was 40 milligrams of aescin three times per day for up to two months. A typical dose of horse chestnut is 250 milligrams (corresponding to 100 milligrams of aescin) two times a day with meals.

Libido

Libido exists on a spectrum: some folks have a higher libido as their natural state while others naturally run at a lower speed. Even for the same person over time, different periods of life may bring factors that either boost and ignite or dampen and tamp down libido. The medical establishment has tried to establish with certainty what constitutes a healthy libido for diagnostic purposes. But this may be as tricky as trying to define what constitutes a "good" sex life. Is it the number of times you have sex, or is it rather more about the quality, presence, and orgasmic potential of your sexual interactions?

A healthy libido, like a healthy sex life, will take many different forms for different folks and will probably vary over time. Still, if you're currently experiencing low libido or a lack of sexual desire that you wish to address and revive, herbs can help. Common causes of low libido include physiological factors like hormonal imbalance, postpartum, use of the contraceptive pill, certain medications, chronic pelvic pain, orgasmic dysfunction, and pain with intercourse. Other possible causes of low libido include a lack of Eros in life, being stuck in a rut or a dull routine, and a lack of foreplay or other sensual stimulation.

Libido and hormonal balance go hand in hand. Common culprits for low libido include an overload of cortisol, also known as the stress hormone. High cortisol levels decrease arousal and desire and lower satisfaction in the sexual function index.[66] Adaptogen herbs like ashwagandha and maca regulate the stress response and increase the body's resistance to stress by keeping cortisol levels in check. Ashwagandha root, for example, has been studied in a sixty-day prospective, double-blind, randomized, placebo-controlled trial to assess its stress-reducing and cortisol regulating effect.[67] The results show a marked reduction in serum cortisol levels in the ashwagandha group compared with the placebo group. The dosage was a 300-milligram capsule of concentrated ashwagandha root extract twice daily.

Aside from stress hormones, a well-functioning thyroid is also essential for healthy libido. Low levels of thyroid hormone are associated with low libido, among other symptoms like fatigue and weight gain. Here, ashwagandha root may provide support as well. Ashwagandha root extract improves thyroid function by enhancing thyroid hormones and by preventing the oxidative stress that negatively impacts thyroid health.[68]

Finally, one more type of hormone is intimately connected to healthy libido: the sex hormones estrogen, progesterone, and testosterone. An imbalance in these hormones may cause low libido and sexual desire dysfunction. Medicinal herbs with a balancing effect on sex hormones include ashwagandha root, nettle root, vitex, and maca. In a randomized, double-blind, placebo-controlled, crossover study on the hormonal effects of ashwagandha in overweight men between the ages of forty and seventy, the use of ashwagandha was associated with a 14.7 percent increase in testosterone compared with placebo after eight weeks of treatment.[69] Testosterone is positively associated with a higher libido. The dosage was two 300-milligram tablets of ashwagandha extract once daily for eight weeks.

Life stages such as breast-feeding, postpartum, and menopause can all affect libido for a time. There is no reason to pathologize this hormonal dance that fluctuates and impacts libido as a result. However, for those seeking to boost up their sexual desire and arousal, some herbs may be of assistance. Damiana, maca, and shatavari are powerful aphrodisiacs that also provide nourishment for the body and the nervous system.

Damiana is both an aphrodisiac and an antidepressant nervine. Maca is an adaptogenic aphrodisiac and regulates the stress response. It enhances stamina and energy levels and provides intense nutrition as a nutrient-rich root vegetable loaded with vitamins, minerals, and bioavailable secondary metabolites with a hormone-balancing action. Shatavari is an adaptogenic aphrodisiac as well. It enhances arousal, vaginal wetness, and lubrication. I like to blend them all into a sensual tincture blend, taken daily.

Hormonal contraceptives lower libido and squash desire in some people. For users of the contraceptive pill and other hormonal contraception, the link between hormonal birth control and libido has been well investigated. Hormonal birth control changes sex-hormone-binding globulin (SHBG) levels, decreases circulating androgen levels, lowers the baseline serum levels of estradiol and progesterone, and inhibits the functioning in the body of oxytocin (known as the "love" hormone or the "cuddle" hormone).[70]

Other medications like SSRIs, which are used in the context of depression, are known to impact sex drive as well. They change libido levels by affecting serotonin (the "happy" hormone) and dopamine (the "pleasure and reward" hormone) in the brain. While SSRIs increase the amount of serotonin circulating in the brain, lessening feelings of depression and anxiety, too much serotonin can inhibit sex drive and make it harder to get aroused and experience sexual pleasure.[71]

Another theory on why antidepressants affect sex drive is that as serotonin increases, levels of dopamine may decrease. Because enough dopamine is required in order to feel stimulation, the result of less dopamine is lower libido and less sexual desire.[72] But herbs can help. In an open trial, the circulatory tonic herb *Ginkgo biloba* was found to reverse antidepressant-induced sexual dysfunction with a positive effect on all four phases of the sexual response cycle: desire, excitement, orgasm, and resolution.[73]

Pain in many forms lowers libido and sex drive. For physical pain, turmeric and ginger offer anti-inflammatory pain relief. The herbs dong quai and yarrow provide relief for conditions of chronic pelvic pain that hinder a healthy sex life. In small doses, soothing nervines and antispasmodics like valerian root and California poppy relieve painful spasms and cramping. As for pain in the emotional realm, uplifting herbs like rose, milky oats, damiana, passionflower, and lemon balm all possess beneficial action for liberating the mind from worries and tending to the heart, freeing space to enjoy a healthy and whole-hearted erotic and sensual life.

Lubrication

For people with vaginas, lubrication and libido might be thought of as indispensable partners. The experience of vaginal dryness may be painful to discuss for some folks because it can weave into your view of yourself as desirable and sensual. But lubrication is not automatic, and as with all other bodily processes, it is affected by thoughts, emotions, environment and surroundings, stress levels, and overall health.

There are two important types of sexual lubrication: one is associated with being turned on, and the other is the daily lubrication that simply keeps the vagina and vulva moist and prevents uncomfortable dryness. Aside from making sex painful, chronic dryness from lack of daily lubrication makes simple daily habits like walking and sitting suddenly uncomfortable.

Common causes for chronic vaginal dryness include the phases of the menstrual cycle, for instance during the luteal phase of the menstrual cycle. Higher levels of estrogen during the follicular and ovulatory phase of the cycle assist with juicier and more abundant lubrication compared with other phases of the cycle where the vagina may be drier, like during the luteal phase before menstruation. In terms of lubrication during sexual activity, vaginal dryness can be caused by the lack of foreplay, not enough sensual touching or kindling of erotic thoughts and desires, and not feeling safe, wanted, and desired. And sometimes, no matter how turned on you are, wetness may just not be at the rendezvous.

Other common causes of vaginal dryness include hormonal imbalances. Endocrine dysregulation can lead to a decrease in natural lubrication. Postpartum and breast-feeding also play a role in vaginal dryness because prolactin—one of the hormones responsible for breast milk production—lowers the estrogen levels required to ensure wetness. Similarly, vaginal dryness can be linked to hormonal birth control. The pill, rings and patches, and hormonal intrauterine devices (IUDs) all lower estrogen in the body by mimicking what naturally happens during the luteal phase, which leads to dryness.

Finally, the use of conventional intimate care products like tampons, menstrual pads, scented menstrual products, douches, and sprays can disrupt the vaginal microbiome and lead to chronic vaginal dryness as well. These products commonly contain toxins irritating to the highly permeable vaginal membranes and to the vulva. This list includes dioxins, furans, fragrance, dyes, pesticide residue, and other known endocrine disruptors that don't belong anywhere near your genitals!

Lubricants: Which One Should You Choose?

Having sex while lacking proper lubrication not only makes intercourse uncomfortable; it can result in injury. When the vagina isn't properly lubricated and wet during sex, pain and abrasions can result and lead to irritation and inflammation, chronic yeast and bacterial infections, and increased likelihood of sexually transmitted infections. Don't be shy to use lube liberally during sexual play—it's wise, healthy, and sexy. But conventional lubricants carry their own set of risks and are best avoided. Not only do they contain toxic ingredients, they also cause inflammation in the vagina and anus. They can disrupt cellular turnover, elasticity, and pH balance.

Lubes typically come in three categories: oil-based (which is incompatible with condoms), water-based, and silicone-based. The use of water-based over-the-counter personal lubricants can dry out and irritate vaginal and rectal tissue, resulting in dryness, burning, irritation, microbial imbalance, and infection.[74] A 2008 study on the popular commercial lubricants Femglide, K-Y Jelly, and Astroglide demonstrated tissue damage in the vagina that ranged from moderate to severe as a direct result of their use.[75] Intimate wellness is built upon a complex and delicate interplay between the biochemistry and microbiome of the vagina, and this fine-tuned dance is worth protecting. Products formulated with little care and chock-full of disruptive ingredients are best avoided in your bedroom.

Common ingredients in conventional oil-based lubes run the gamut from petroleum and petroleum-derived oils, which coat the vaginal tissues and are associated with an increased risk of bacterial vaginosis (BV). Petroleum-based products may be contaminated with polycyclic aromatic hydrocarbons (PAHs), which are a byproduct of the manufacturing process and to which cancer, persistence, bioaccumulation, and endocrine disruption are all strongly associated.

Silicone-based lubes, on the other hand, coat the vaginal walls and the vulva, making it slippery and silky—but with a price. Silicone may interfere with healthy vaginal function by disrupting pH, microbiome balance, and tissue health.

Other problematic ingredients in lube include propylene glycol, parabens, synthetic fragrances, and spermicides like nonoxynol-9. Herbalist and author of *Hot Pants: Do-It-Yourself Gynecology and Herbal Remedies* Isabelle Gauthier shares a cautionary tale about this particular spermicide:

"The problem is that it's a little too strong. I once watched an Australian sex worker use a single condom lubricated with nonoxynol-9 to remove nail polish off both her hands."[76] Use with caution!

Three ingredients stand out as safe and pleasurable options for luscious lubing: pure aloe vera gel, vegetable glycerin, and coconut oil. Aloe vera gel and vegetable glycerin are condom-safe, while coconut oil is not. Aloe vera and vegetable glycerin are compatible with one another, which means you can easily blend the two at a half-and-half ratio, or another ratio of your choosing. Coconut oil can be used in its natural form (hard at cooler temperature, and liquid at warmer temperature). In cold northern climates, you may opt for fractionated coconut oil, which stays liquid and is easier to play with during sex.

Herbal Lubes

Herbal lubes blend the benefits of herbs together with natural lube ingredients like vegetable glycerin and coconut oil. Vegetable glycerin has been suspected of contributing to vaginal yeast infections for some due to its natural sugars. But if that's a concern to you, you can infuse your vegetable glycerin with healing antifungal herbs like calendula. The antifungal and anticandida activity of calendula has been observed in many studies. In a 2008 Brazilian study, calendula was effective against all twenty-three fungus strains tested.[77]

Another study confirmed similar results, where calendula tincture showed potent antifungal activity against all eight of the yeasts tested.[78] Calendula is as effective as standard antibiotics in fighting yeast and candida, with none of the associated side effects. Calendula is a soothing herb with many benefits to mucosa and vaginal and anal tissues. A calendula glycerite mixed with a dollop of pure aloe vera gel makes for a perfect lubricant that won't harm vaginal balance or disrupt its ecology. Glycerin-based herbal lubes are condom-friendly.

For oil-based herbal lubes, calendula can also be extracted in liquid coconut oil. Other herbs well suited to oil extraction for lube-making include plantain leaf—a soothing anti-inflammatory herb with benefit to mucosa and the vaginal and anal lining—as well as shatavari root, which has a strong affinity with the female sexual organs. Oil- and cacao butter–based lubricants are not compatible with latex condoms.

Wetness Herbs

Taken internally in the form of capsules or tinctures, shatavari root increases lubrication and wetness. Two of shatavari's active constituents are shatavarin and sarsasapogenin, which are potent precursors to female sex hormones. For the purpose of enhancing libido and wetness, shatavari should be ingested regularly. Take shatavari for at least two to three weeks and preferably longer for best results. A safe adaptogen herb, shatavari can be taken safely over long periods. Take it in tincture form, in powders added to warm drinks, or in capsules.

Many other herbs aside from shatavari have also been studied for their benefit to vaginal cells and enhanced lubrication for wellness and sexual health.[79] Dong quai, vitex, wild yam, black cohosh, ginseng, and licorice exert significant benefit to the health of the vaginal lining, which creates a solid (yet silky, slippery, and super wet) foundation for sexual and reproductive wellness to spring from.

Menopause

Menopause is not a health condition nor a pathology: it is simply a normal life passage that all people with female reproductive systems will experience when they reach the end of their reproductive years. Symptoms of discomfort associated with the transition of menopause include hot flashes, night sweats that affect sleep quality, fatigue, vaginal dryness, irritability and mood swings, depression, and other symptoms shared by countless women.

Because menopause as a life passage has been underresearched and often pathologized, many medical therapies have sprouted with an aim to "fix" menopause. The buzz of hormone replacement therapy (HRT), for example, reached a feverish high when renowned endocrinologists in the 1960s and 1970s redefined menopause as an "estrogen-deficiency disease" rather than a normal biological process. When the risks of injecting estrogen over long periods came to light—such as increased risk of endometrial cancer—the hormone progesterone was then added to the hormone replacement therapy regimen, and what was known as estrogen-deficiency disease was soon rebranded as "hormone deficiency syndrome."

More medical therapies for fixing menopause symptoms include surgical interventions like hysterectomies or the total removal of the uterus (and often the ovaries as well), which have been suggested to menopausal women as a way to fix their pelvic health symptoms. Finally, menopausal women are likely to be prescribed antidepressants to address their emotional and mental symptoms associated with this important life transition.

While medical and psychiatric treatment may be of help to some menopausal women, many are looking to reclaim this stage of life and are seeking to embrace it with the help of natural herbal remedies. Many of the conventional treatments for menopausal symptoms hinder sexual health and function. But for women looking to keep their sexual wellness and vibrancy alive, herbs offer a healthful alternative.

What Happens During Menopause?

As menopause nears, the ovaries gradually start producing less estrogen. Eventually, the ovaries stop releasing eggs as well. Menstruation becomes more erratic until it stops altogether. You know you've entered full menopause when you haven't had a menstruation in over twelve consecutive months. Altered hormone levels that come from the end of the reproductive years can cause unpleasant symptoms like hot flashes, mood swings, irritability, brain fog, fatigue, and low libido. Medicinal herbs are widely used to support hormonal health during menopause. Herbal allies for menopausal women include black cohosh, vitex, dong quai, maca, and sage.

Black cohosh is used by many women to treat menopausal problems. It is effective in reducing hot flashes and night sweats. In a 2018 study with eighty menopausal women who experienced hot flashes, black cohosh significantly reduced the severity and frequency of hot flashes and improved quality of life.[80]

In another recent study, black cohosh was shown to be more effective and much safer than the conventional menopausal hormone therapy drug tibolone, which is used for fibroids, endometriosis, and osteoporosis.[81] Black cohosh was more effective than conventional treatment in shrinking fibroid size and preventing their growth. Fibroids are one of the most common reasons leading menopausal women to seek hysterectomies.

The benefits of black cohosh for menopausal women don't stop there. Black cohosh also helps increase the quality of sleep in women undergoing menopause. Finally, there were no adverse reactions measured in women who received a daily administration of black cohosh over a six-month period.[82] Their liver function, kidney function, and pelvic and breast health were monitored, with no negative changes found. Despite some claims that black cohosh may increase the risk of breast cancer, a systematic review of scientific literature has found no correlation between use of black cohosh and increased breast cancer risk.[83] Use black cohosh in tincture form, in capsules, or as part of an herbal blend with other botanicals.

Vitex, also known as chaste tree or chasteberry, is a supreme herbal ally of women in their menopausal years. In a 2019 randomized, controlled, double-blind clinical trial with a study group of fifty-two menopausal women, vitex exerted significant benefit in the relief of night sweats, hot flashes, vaginal dryness, heart palpitations, and other vasomotor symptoms, along with significant relief from anxiety compared with the placebo group.[84] After eight weeks of follow-up and at the end of study, the results of the comparison between the vitex and placebo groups regarding the mean scores of menopausal complications demonstrated that vitex had exerted benefit to all menopausal complications tested in the study. Each one!

Vitex extract is an inexpensive, effective, and safe treatment with no side effects that can be applied as a nonhormonal remedy option along with other therapy methods available for menopausal complications. Herbal tradition supports the use of vitex for menopausal complaints. So do pharmacological studies and clinical research rooted in the endocrinology and neuroendocrinology of menopause and associated symptoms.[85] Use vitex as a tincture or in capsule form.

Dong quai is a popular staple of Traditional Chinese Medicine and a beloved female tonic herb. In a randomized controlled trial comparing a combined preparation of dong quai and chamomile to placebo among fifty-five women reporting hot flashes and refusing hormone therapy, the herbal blend demonstrated clinically significant improvement in the frequency and intensity of hot flashes (90–96 percent) compared with placebo (15–20 percent) over the three-month trial.[86] Dong quai can be taken in tincture form or in capsules.

In a double-blind, placebo-controlled, randomized controlled trial, dong quai was combined with black cohosh, milk thistle, red clover, American ginseng, and vitex and tested among fifty healthy women.[87] At twelve weeks, participants receiving the herbal preparation reported a 73 percent reduction in hot flashes and a 69 percent decrease in night sweats, compared with 38 percent and 29 percent improvement in the placebo group, respectively.

Maca is an adaptogen herb from Peru. Maca root supports the endocrine and reproductive systems. It boosts the production of sex hormones and increases energy along with sex drive. In studies, maca supplementation was associated with a substantial reduction of menopausal discomfort in early postmenopausal women. A 2005 double-blind, placebo-corrected clinical pilot study on the effects of maca for menopausal complaints demonstrated maca's ability to substantially reduce menopausal discomfort and symptoms.[88] The dosage used was two 500-milligram hard-gel capsules twice daily.

A 2008 study on maca also showed that maca alleviates symptoms of anxiety and depression while boosting libido and sexual function in postmenopausal women.[89] Because of the high safety profile of maca, which is safe when taken in recommended doses over long periods, I recommend that menopausal women give maca a try when they experience menopausal complaints.

Sage is an aromatic botanical used to alleviate hot flashes, sweating, and other menopausal symptoms as a general tonic. A 2019 study on the effects of sage on postmenopausal women showed that sage reduces the severity of hot flashes, lowers the occurrence of night sweats, lessens episodes of panic and fatigue, and enhances concentration and focus.[90] The participants, all women between the ages of forty-six and fifty-eight, received a 100-milligram capsule of sage extract daily for four weeks.

Traditional use and science both recognize the value of sage as an herbal extract for menopause. An open, multicenter clinical trial in Switzerland in 2011 found that sage extract helped the mean number of mild, moderate, severe, and very severe hot flashes to decrease by 46 percent, 62 percent, 79 percent, and 100 percent over eight weeks, respectively.[91] The treatment was well tolerated with no reported side effects.

For women crossing the bridge to menopause, herbs can act as allies and companions along the way. Nervines and antidepressants like California poppy and damiana are of great support for mood-lifting and relieving irritability. Psychotropic herbs like kava and blue lotus, along with cannabis and psilocybin mushrooms, might also be beneficial for women seeking a different pace of life, one that may continue to guide the wisdom of your elder years as priorities shift and as your body, mind, heart, and psyche undergo transformation.

Menstrual Cycle

An intimate understanding of the menstrual cycle is essential both for family planning and natural contraception, as well as for optimal conception and pregnancy. Girls and young women undergoing menarche, or the beginning of their menstrual cycle, also benefit from a better connection to their bodies and natural rhythms as they enter their reproductive years. The same goes for perimenopausal and menopausal women who stand on the other end of their reproductive journey.

Aside from fertility awareness, there are many other benefits to tuning in to the menstrual cycle. Healing conditions like irregular cycles, heavy bleeding or spotting, PMS, menstrual cramps, menstrual migraines, and hormonal imbalances rests on the ability to tune in to the hormonal cycles unfolding inside the body. Finally, gaining a better understanding of inner rhythm helps guide days and creative projects.

Common conditions associated with the menstrual cycle include dysmenorrhea (menstrual pain and cramping, ranging from moderate to severe), anovulation (no ovulation), and amenorrhea (lack of menstrua-tion). Herbal remedies and medicinal herbs have a long history as allies for menstrual health conditions.

The Four Phases of the Menstrual Cycle

The menstrual cycle includes the uterine cycle and the ovarian cycle. Together, they are divided into four distinct phases: menstruation, the fol-licular phase, ovulation, and the luteal phase. The first day of menstruation (bleeding, not spotting) marks the beginning of the menstrual cycle. This day also signals the start of the follicular phase, which lasts about fourteen days or more, or until the day of ovulation.

Ovulation is instantly followed by the luteal phase, which leads to menstruation and the start of a new menstrual cycle. Menstrual bleeding can last from three to eight days. Whole menstrual cycle length does vary from body to body, and for the same person over time. The menstrual cycle may last twenty-one to forty days, with an overall average of twenty-eight days. Even though a twenty-eight-day cycle has been hailed as the standard number of days in the medical literature, it is not the menstrual holy grail that folks should aim for.

My own menstrual cycle has been exactly twenty-five days long ever since I started menstruating about twenty years ago. My bleeding time lasts four days. One of my good friends, on the other hand, has a cycle length of thirty-five days and bleeds for eight or nine days. Both cycles (and women) are healthy.

The menstrual cycle is regulated by the ovaries, uterus, brain (hypo-thalamus and pituitary), thyroid gland, and adrenal glands. Balance and interconnectedness are the name of the game here. The adrenals commu-nicate with the ovaries and the thyroid. The thyroid communicates back to the ovaries. This cyclical feedback loop builds the foundation on which the menstrual cycle rests. As with other bodily cycles, the dance of reproduc-tive hormones that guides the ebb and flow of the menstrual cycle phases can be disrupted by stress, toxins, oppression, and other concerns.

Today, it is a rarity that a woman's menstrual cycle functions optimally throughout the reproductive years—it is rare and no longer the norm.

After all, the endocrine system governs the release of the reproductive hormones that are responsible for a healthy menstrual cycle. Endocrine disruptors in the environment, along with stress overload and other factors, make the work of the endocrine system extra tough to handle. That's why I recommend endocrine tonics—adaptogens—as well as liver tonics to my herbal clients whenever they want to address menstrual conditions. This helps regulate the hormones involved in menstrual wellness. The hormones responsible for orchestrating the four phases of the menstrual cycle include luteinizing hormone (LH), follicle-stimulating hormone (FSH), estrogen, and progesterone.

Follicular and Luteal: What's the Difference?

The follicular phase, or the first half of the menstrual cycle when estrogen is highest, is when an egg grows and develops. It is marked by higher energy levels, is more outward focused, and with libido rising until ovulation, when it is at its highest. Women at this time feel attractive, personable, energetic, sensual, and caring. For folks who do cycle charting with basal body temperature, temps range from 97°F to 97.5°F. Cervical mucus is slippery, stretchy, and wet.

The luteal phase, or second half of the menstrual cycle when progesterone is highest, is marked by a stronger desire for rest and is more inward focused, with inner reflection and emotions rising. Women at this time feel more in tune with their feelings, frustrations, and unmet needs. On the other hand, the progesterone boost might also bring feelings of serenity, deep contentment, and tranquility. The luteal phase happens before menstruation and is often a time when women experience premenstrual syndrome or PMS. Basal body temps go slightly higher than in the previous phase and reach 97.5°F to 98.6°F. Cervical mucus is sticky, creamy, or dry.

A Note on Menstrual Products

Conventional tampons and menstrual pads are harmful to health. They are not manufactured with women's best interests and comfort in mind. Menstrual care products are made with a toxic slew of chemicals, many of which can be absorbed into the bloodstream via the vaginal walls. In 2014, a women's organization sent menstrual products for laboratory testing.[92] Four types of menstrual pads manufactured by Procter & Gamble under the brand name Always were analyzed for traces of volatile organic compounds. The results showed problematic amounts of many chemicals, including styrene (a carcinogen), chloromethane (a reproductive toxicant), chloroethane (a carcinogen), chloroform (a carcinogen, reproductive toxicant, and neurotoxin), and acetone (an irritant).

A 2019 study published in *Reproductive Toxicology* demonstrated similar results.[93] Researchers found that phthalate concentrations in the eleven brands of sanitary pads tested were significantly higher than usual concentrations found in common commercial plastic products, which are harmful to begin with. This is of particular concern because sanitary pads are in direct contact with the genitals for an extended period. As such, it's likely that a considerable amount of volatile organic compounds and phthalates are absorbed into the reproductive system.

It is a true sign of pervasive sexism that women's care products—essential products—have been allowed to be profoundly toxic and harmful to health with no regulations or government oversight holding manufacturers and companies accountable. As part of my herbal practice, I advise my herbal clients who seek to regulate and optimize their menstrual cycle to avoid conventional menstrual products as part of their menstrual wellness protocol. Instead, I recommend using menstrual cups or washable and reusable cotton pads.

Amenorrhea: Menstruation Gone Missing

Amenorrhea is the absence of menstruation. It affects people with uteruses for a variety of reasons, such as a low body weight, caloric restriction, extreme dietary restriction, overexercising, stress, and endocrine imbalances. At an ashram in the Bahamas where I stayed for a winter when I was twenty years old, I met many women who had stopped menstruating as a result of their sattvic diet, a type of repetitive yogic diet that was followed at that ashram. In this case, it was also a vegan diet. *Sattvic* comes from the Sanskrit word *sattva* in the Vedic philosophy and translates as "pure" and "wholesome." Clearly, it wasn't that wholesome if it resulted in women losing their periods!

When they found out I was an herbalist and women's health practitioner, they asked for some advice on getting their periods back. I happened to have Queen Anne's lace seeds with me, in large quantities, because I was using it as birth control at the time (my partner and I were game for asana, but not *brahmacharya*—no sexual abstinence for us, thank you very much!). This is purely anecdotal, but a few women at the ashram started menstruating after consuming Queen Anne's lace tea. I reasoned it was probably due to the seeds' tonifying effect on the uterus that helped expel old stagnant blood and move stuck womb energy, resulting in menstrual flow.

Menstrual Cycle and PMS

Premenstrual syndrome (PMS) affects up to 80 percent of menstruating women. The symptoms of PMS range from mild to severe and debilitating. Irritability, mood swings, bloating and digestive discomfort, menstrual migraines, cramps, diarrhea, nausea and vomiting, and an uptick in arthritic or joint pain and inflammation are all possible symptoms of PMS.

While PMS is often attributed to hormonal imbalances, common symptoms of PMS may actually be caused by a variety of factors. Nutrient deficiencies, stress, adrenal fatigue, endocrine dysregulation, sexism, cultural period shaming, discomfort with emotions like sadness and anger, and a lack of body literacy can all contribute to PMS symptoms as well.

Period pain (dysmenorrhea) in the lower pelvic area is a common PMS symptom. It is associated with an excess of prostaglandins, the inflammatory chemicals responsible for uterine spasms and cramping. Medicinal herbs can be of great help for PMS prevention and management. Beneficial herbs include antispasmodics like valerian to relieve pain and cramping, calming and mood-lifting nervines like passionflower to soothe irritability and anxiety, and hormone balancers like maca and vitex to regulate the cycle.

Valerian root is a potent antispasmodic. Valerian relieves painful uterine spasms and cramping. Because valerian offers relief both physically, mentally, and emotionally, it is a great herbal choice for those who experience severe PMS. As a sedative, valerian in high doses will make you sleepy and support deep rest. I recommend valerian root tincture for this purpose, taken as needed.

Passionflower is a calming and mood-lifting herb beneficial for the nervous system. Passionflower helps those who find themselves cranky, moody, and irritable during their premenstrual period. Passionflower may be of special assistance to folks who tend to cry and be weepy as a mark of PMS. For best results, take passionflower daily in capsule form or tincture.

Maca root is an adaptogen, endocrine regulator, and hormone balancer. Maca regulates the menstrual cycle and provides relief from PMS. It exerts a balancing action on sex hormone levels. Maca powder can be enjoyed with cacao as a nourishing drink.

Vitex berry is a regulator of the hormone cycle via balancing progesterone and estrogen throughout the menstrual cycle. Vitex is specifically indicated for high estrogen conditions like endometriosis, uterine fibroids, and ovarian cysts. PMS symptoms that call for vitex are swollen breasts, breast tenderness, anxiety, stress, and tension. For best results, take vitex tincture or capsules throughout the menstrual cycle.

Cramp bark is a beneficial antispasmodic used for menstrual cramping. Cramp bark relaxes the uterine muscle and prevents muscular spasms. Use it for uterine cramps as well as ovarian cramps. Take cramp bark tincture as needed when cramps arise.

Ginger is a warming spice that alleviates menstrual pain and aches. Ginger brings warmth and relief to lower-back pain and pain in the pelvic area radiating down the legs. Healing aromatic ginger also prevents the increase in arthritic pain or chronic pain that can worsen before menstruation. Anti-inflammatory, pain-relieving, and antiemetic, ginger relieves the nausea and vomiting associated with intense period pain. My favorite way to enjoy ginger for this purpose is ginger candies or ginger glycerite, taken as needed.

Menstrual Cycle and Estrogen Dominance

Estrogen is essential for maintaining fertility, immune function, healthy bones, cardiovascular health, and blood sugar balance. Too much estrogen, however, can cause many unwanted symptoms and lead to menstrual problems. Signs of estrogen excess include a short follicular phase, heavy bright-red bleeding during menstruation, chin acne around ovulation, swollen and sensitive breasts, fibrocystic breasts, fibroids, weight gain, and hypothyroid symptoms like cold hands and feet.

Estrogen dominance is becoming a widespread issue. Many functional doctors associate estrogen excess to the presence of xenoestrogens in the environment and in consumer products like furniture and clothing. Xenoestrogens are chemicals that mimic estrogen in the body. Aside from avoiding xenoestrogens and other endocrine disruptors, the best way to guard against and reverse estrogen dominance is by enhancing liver function, detoxification, and elimination.

Yarrow leaf and flower is a nice bitter herb with hepatic properties. It supports liver detoxification functions, which are essential to hormonal balance and the processing of excess hormones like estrogen. Enjoy it as a tincture or an infusion.

Milk thistle seed is a supreme liver remedy. Milk thistle is extensively used and researched for its liver-protective abilities. Herbalists use milk thistle as a hepatic trophorestorative, commonly in the form of a tincture or capsule. Milk thistle is especially useful in the context of estrogen dominance. It will enhance estrogen clearance from the body and improves phase 1 and phase 2 liver detox.

Milk thistle seed is such a powerful liver tonic that it is used to help reverse mushroom poisoning from the deadly death cap mushroom (*Amanita phalloides*). A concentrated extract from milk thistle called silibinin, when administered intravenously to folks who have consumed death cap mushroom and are on their potential deathbed, prevents hepatic failure, reduces the need for liver transplant, and lowers the death rate from liver poisoning.[94]

Turmeric root, the golden spice, offers antioxidant and anti-inflammatory properties. As a liver tonic, turmeric enhances liver function and supports detoxification. Daily intake of turmeric or curcumin ensures proper estrogen clearance and protects against hormonal imbalance.

Schisandra berry is a classic herbal remedy of Traditional Chinese Medicine. Schisandra offers support to the female reproductive system while also being a potent liver tonic. This makes schisandra a strong ally in all things related to hormonal imbalance and the relative ratio of estrogen to progesterone. It is an adaptogen and aphrodisiac. I love schisandra tincture and recommend it to most of my clients, taken daily.

Menstrual Cycle and Heavy Bleeding

For heavy menstrual bleeding, important herbs include styptics to stop the excessive vaginal bleeding as well as nutritive iron-rich herbs to replenish nutrient stores that get depleted in the process. Note that for anyone experiencing heavy menstrual bleeding, it is recommended that you work with your health care provider to uncover the cause. Sometimes heavy bleeding can be caused by other factors, like fibroids or hormonal imbalances, that need to be addressed and may not be supported by styptic herbs and nutritive herbs alone.

Styptic herbs include yarrow and shepherd's purse. Yarrow is a uterine tonic and stimulant. It balances blood flow. Use it for excessive menstrual bleeding lasting more than eight days or totaling more than 80 milliliters of blood volume. Shepherd's purse is a styptic and hemostatic herb and is often combined with yarrow in the form of a tincture for heavy menstrual bleeding, taken as needed.

Nettle is an iron-rich nutritive tonic herb especially beneficial for heavy bleeding during menstruation. In cases of heavy bleeding that results in fatigue, nettle is recommended throughout the cycle as a nutrient booster. It is rich in calcium, magnesium, and other minerals and vitamins that relieve PMS symptoms linked with nutrient deficiencies. Take nettle as a nourishing infusion.

Menstrual Migraines

Many women suffer from regular menstrual migraines and frontal headaches that are cyclical in nature and associated with fluctuating hormones.

Though herbs don't offer quick pain relief for menstrual migraines, herbal remedies address the root cause of the issue and reverse the condition in the long term. A blend of adaptogen herbs along with liver tonics work wonders on menstrual migraines. Excellent liver tonic herbs in this context include schisandra, turmeric, and milk thistle.

Clinical experience shows that the Japanese remedy tokishakuyakusan (TSS), known as danggui shaoyao san in Traditional Chinese Medicine, is highly effective in the treatment of menstrual migraines.[95] This remedy contains dong quai and peony root. In one study, five female patients ranging in age from twenty to forty-eight were successfully relieved of their chronic menstrual migraines following treatment with dong quai and peony root. The dosage used was 2.5 grams of herbal extract twice per day. Pain relief was apparent after only one month of treatment, and there were no reported side effects.

Menstrual Cycle and Fertility

A little-known fact about women's biology and the menstrual cycle is that women only have five to ten days per month when they can become pregnant. The day of ovulation, when one of the ovaries releases an egg, is in fact the only fertile time throughout the menstrual cycle. But the five to ten days or so leading up to ovulation are also considered to be a part of the fertile window because sperm can hang around for a while, ready to pounce at the first sign of an egg missile.

For the folks who want to avoid pregnancy, this means that you'll want to abstain from penetrative sex or that you'll use protection during the fertile window in order to prevent conception from taking place around ovulation. On the flip side, for those who want to optimize their chances of conceiving a baby during the fertile window, this is the time when you want to be having lots of juicy orgasmic sex.

The best way to know for sure when ovulation occurs is to practice cycle charting. If cycles are irregular, ovulation may take place at random times and be harder to predict effectively, impacting fertility and conception. That's why hormone regulating herbs are helpful in balancing the menstrual cycle and supporting your cyclic flow.

One more note about the menstrual cycle and fertility: many of my friends in their early thirties who are now actively trying to start their families have become masters at cycle charting, regulating their cycles, and pinpointing exactly when they ovulate. But there is one problem they encounter smack-dab in the middle of their fertile window—they're just too darn tired for sex. Swamped, drained, exhausted, sleepy, not in the mood; you name it. Tiredness clearly has an impact on your ability to get in the mood for sex. What's more, I hear from many people who think that "planning" sex during their fertile window is, well, unsexy (it's not).

In any case, herbs can help. Adaptogens like maca, shatavari, and ashwagandha all bring benefit to stress regulation and energy balance. Uplifting nervines like damiana and milky oats support the getting-in-the-mood part of sexual wellness. There's no shame in needing a bit of help in that department. And besides, as famed relationship therapist Esther Perel has taught us, scheduling and planning intentional sex doesn't have to take away the spontaneous erotic spark—far from it. Making a shared commitment to cycle charting, to fertility herbs, to aphrodisiacs, and to making time for sexual connection is an act of pleasure-centered liberation and empowerment.

Cycle Charting

Understanding and knowing the menstrual cycle in an intimate way is a step toward reproductive freedom and the reappropriation of the body and its natural rhythms. One way to better understand the rhythms of the menstrual cycle is through cycle charting. Cycle charting can be done with the calendar method, complete with tracking your basal body temperature, cervical fluids, and cervix shape and location. Cycle charting involves keeping track of your menstrual cycle data month after month to observe patterns or a lack thereof. It might be helpful to keep a small yearly calendar or daily planner on hand for this purpose, or find an app. Write down any bodily symptom, emotion, time when you started bleeding, color of the blood, presence of clotting, changes in libido, and more.

In my practice, I recommend cycle charting to all of my menstruating clients. It offers them a personal and intimate view into their rhythms. Many find it to be empowering and liberating. I've heard various folks report having had a bad experience with cycle charting apps (leading to false or incorrect cycle assessments, poor predictions, or inconclusive reports). If that's happened to you, don't despair and ditch cycle charting. Instead, ditch your smartphone and apps. A good old pen and calendar does the trick better than any algorithm. The benefits of cycle charting ripple back to health practitioners as well and are worth adding to your practice. As a practitioner, my clients' cycle charts offer an invaluable window into their current reproductive rhythms and flow.

Cycle charting helps assess follicular phase length, luteal phase length, the occurrence of ovulation, possible anovulation, hormonal balance between estrogen and progesterone, and when conception occurs. When you cycle-chart, and if pregnancy occurs, you'll know exactly what day you conceived. For best results with your cycle charting, track your basal body temperature (BBT), cervical fluids, and cervical changes.

Tracking Basal Body Temperature (BBT)

This is done by taking your oral temperature with an under-the-tongue thermometer every morning upon waking. Once a full monthly cycle of temperature charting has been completed, you will notice that the follicular phase is marked by slightly cooler temperature (97°F to 97.5°F), while the luteal phase is marked by slightly hotter temperature (97.5°F to 98.6°F). This is called the biphasic shift. Tracking your BBT over time will enable you to pinpoint exactly on which day you ovulate. The temperature spike signals that you've ovulated. In that way, it doesn't predict ovulation but rather shows that it happened in the previous twenty-four hours. Throughout the months, you'll be able to establish on which day you typically ovulate, for prediction purposes. For example, I usually ovulate on day 14 of my menstrual cycle.

Tracking Cervical Fluids

Cervical fluids have a different flow, color, consistency, and texture depending on which phase of the menstrual cycle you find yourself in. In the days following menstruation, the vagina might be drier, which signals you're less fertile. As ovulation approaches, vaginal secretions ramp up and get clear, slippery, and super stretchy, which means it's peak fertility time.

Tracking Cervical Changes

During ovulation, the cervix is higher up in the vagina and softer to the touch.

PCOS and Ovarian Cysts

Polycystic ovary syndrome (PCOS) is one of the most common endocrine reproductive disorders affecting women of childbearing age. PCOS is a common hormonal condition affecting the ovaries and reproductive system. But unlike the name suggests, PCOS is not just a condition of cyst formation in the ovaries; rather, it is a complex endocrine and metabolic disorder affecting ovarian function. Symptoms of PCOS can include ovarian cysts, but you can still have PCOS even if you have no cysts on your ovaries.

PCOS is characterized by obesity, insulin resistance and blood sugar instability, elevated androgen production and high testosterone, increased risk of cardiovascular disease, and imbalance of the hypothalamic-pituitary-adrenal (HPA) axis. Other symptoms of PCOS are menstrual irregularities. This includes infrequent or erratic cycles, less than nine menstrual periods per year (or more than thirty-five days between periods), and heavy bleeding.

Substantial weight gain, along with marked difficulty losing weight no matter what you do, is another hallmark of PCOS, as is excess facial and body hair (hirsutism). PCOS can disrupt women's lives and carries myriad possible complications such as infertility, type 2 diabetes, and mood disorders like depression and anxiety.

There's a strong link between polycystic ovary syndrome and insulin resistance, which affects as many as 65 to 70 percent of women with PCOS. Insulin is the pancreas-made hormone that enables your cells to use sugar (glucose) as energy for the body. If your cells become insulin-resistant, your blood sugar levels will climb, causing your body to produce even more insulin. Excess insulin is linked with androgen production and the type of ovulatory dysfunction so common in PCOS.

PCOS also has a strong association with metabolic syndrome. The numbers don't lie: women with PCOS are up to eleven times more likely to suffer from metabolic syndrome than those without PCOS. Common medical advice teaches that being overweight is a risk factor for metabolic syndrome, as is lack of exercise. But mounting scientific evidence is pointing toward air pollution as a main cause of metabolic syndrome. In a long-term study published in 2021, air pollutants were strongly associated with increased risk of developing the condition.[96] Living with metabolic syndrome increases your risk of cardiovascular disease and atherosclerosis and makes you more vulnerable to insulin resistance, type 2 diabetes, and endometrial cancer.[97]

Chronic low-grade inflammation is a key contributor to PCOS. Inflammation can encourage higher androgen production as well as insulin resistance, leading to weight gain and disrupting the balance of sex hormones responsible for regulating the menstrual cycle. What's more, this type of inflammation is also a feature of conditions like metabolic syndrome, type 2 diabetes, and cardiovascular disease, which are closely associated with PCOS. If you're noticing a looping trail of symptoms that all seem to be contributing to one another, you're right. This is what happens with PCOS.

Studies done in the United States show that, while PCOS affects women of all races and backgrounds, Hispanic women present the most severe PCOS conditions,[98] and Black women with PCOS are significantly more at risk of developing metabolic syndrome and cardiovascular disease compared with White women with PCOS.[99]

When addressing the symptoms and root causes of PCOS with herbs, the focus is on hormonal imbalance, insulin resistance, metabolic syndrome, and chronic low-grade inflammation. Herbal recommendations for PCOS include anti-inflammatory herbs, adaptogens, hepatic tonics, and nervines.

Modern science agrees with the traditional use of medicinal herbs as support for PCOS. Thorough and comprehensive studies show that herbal medicines are promising resources in the development of effective therapeutic agents for the treatment of PCOS.[100] Other preclinical and clinical studies provide evidence that specific herbal medicines have beneficial impacts on women with PCOS and PCOS-related amenorrhea and hyperandrogenism (excess of androgen hormones).[101]

Endocrine outcomes from herbal medicine include reduced luteinizing hormone (LH), lower prolactin, lower fasting insulin, and reduced testosterone—all excellent news in the context of PCOS. The herbs tested include milk thistle, turmeric, black cohosh, and vitex. With the herbs tested, there was evidence for improved ovulatory function, better metabolic hormone profile, and higher fertility outcomes in women with PCOS treated with medicinal herbs. And finally, this should be shouted from the rooftops: there was evidence that two herbs in particular were equivalent to (or, if you consider the herbs' safety profiles, better than) conventional drugs in the treatment of PCOS. The two herbs in question are vitex and black cohosh.

The female tonic herb vitex helps lower prolactin levels. According to naturopathic physician Jill Stansbury, prolactin is typically elevated in women with PCOS and is a leading cause of amenorrhea (lack of menstruation) and infertility.[102] Elevated prolactin can suppress follicle maturation and ovulation and contribute to ovarian cysts. This makes vitex an excellent herbal remedy in the context of PCOS. Vitex also regulates the menstrual cycle and reverses infertility in women with PCOS.

A fascinating study shows that vitex supplementation lengthens a short luteal phase in women with PCOS and short luteal phase defect (which negatively impacts fertility).[103] Luteal phase length increased from a low 3.4 days to a staggering 10.5 days in only three months of treatment with vitex. The dosage was 20 milligrams per day.

Black cohosh lowers luteinizing hormone (LH) levels and increases fertility in women with PCOS. In a study analyzing the effects of black cohosh paired with Clomid (a fertility drug), positive interactions were demonstrated by the addition of black cohosh to the Clomid treatment.[104] In fact, the black cohosh and Clomid group had more than double (43.3 percent) the pregnancy rates compared with the Clomid-only group (20.3 percent). The dosage used was 20 milligrams of black cohosh daily.

In a separate study, the effects of black cohosh versus Clomid were tested for hormone concentrations as well as for pregnancy rates.[105] The black cohosh–only group had better outcomes than the Clomid-only group. In other words, black cohosh is more effective and much safer than conventional drugs for women with PCOS.

A holistic herbal treatment for PCOS includes hormonal herbs such as maca, vitex, and schisandra. Herbs for insulin resistance include dandelion root, turmeric, and ginger. Devil's club is indicated for better blood sugar regulation as well and is specifically used with folks of indigenous descent. Herbs to prevent metabolic syndrome include dong quai, turmeric, and milk thistle, while herbs to reverse chronic inflammation include turmeric, ginger, and nettle. Jill Stansbury recommends the addition of lemon balm to the PCOS herbal protocol for its ability to reduce elevated prolactin via dopamine activity. Lemon balm is also a beneficial nervine and antidepressant herb. My favorite way to enjoy it is in herbal infusions or glycerites.

Prostate Health

The prostate is a part of the male reproductive system. It is a small chestnut-shaped and walnut-sized gland located in front of the rectum and just below the bladder. The prostate is responsible for producing seminal fluid. This fluid provides nutrients to sperm and acts as a carrier for sperm during an ejaculation. The prostate surrounds the urethra, the tube that carries urine and semen through the penis. It is pleasurable to the touch and is known as the male G-spot. It can be reached inside the anus. Aside from its healthful pleasures, the prostate gland needs to be cared for throughout life because many men experience prostate issues in their elder years—specifically enlarged prostate and prostate cancer. Many therapists assert that regular ejaculations keep the prostate healthy. So do herbs.

An enlarged prostate causes painful urination, urinary urgency, incomplete emptying of the bladder, weak flow of urine, and waking up during the night to pee, and it can lead to urinary incontinence. The condition is known as benign prostate hyperplasia (BPH) and it responds very well to herbs. While BPH is benign, it is certainly a possible precursor to prostate cancer, so an effective herbal intervention is worth committing to.

Lastly, prostate cancer is one of the most common cancers affecting men. Some of my herbal clients, older men who have had prostate cancer and had their prostate surgically removed as a result, have reported sexual issues that affect their life and relationships. For example, erectile dysfunction may occur in men post–prostate cancer treatment. I've witnessed strong benefits from medicinal herbs in these men, and many herbalists agree.

The goal of herbal treatment is manyfold: first, to support prostate health and prevent enlargement and tumors. Second, herbs lower the symptoms of prostate enlargement and reduce the risk of malignancy. Finally, herbs assist with prostate cancer treatment. They enhance the chances of success and remission and provide assistance to men and their sexual health along the way. Top herbs to recommend for prostate health include saw palmetto, nettle, dandelion, red clover, and cleavers.

Studies have shown that Black men with prostate cancer have worse health outcomes than their White counterparts.[106] But when equal-access health care is added to the mix, it turns out that the disparity between races evens out.

Saw palmetto is a primary tonic for the male reproductive system. It supports prostate and urinary tract health, as well as hormonal regulation of testosterone, libido, and sexual potency. Saw palmetto is used to treat genitourinary problems, to enhance sperm production and libido, and as a mild diuretic herb for enhanced urinary output. The prostate gland converts active testosterone into dihydrotestosterone (DHT). DHT is responsible for prostate growth and can lead to problematic enlargement. But saw palmetto along with nettle root inhibit the formation of DHT in the prostate. They accomplish this by blocking the enzyme 5-alpha-reductase that converts testosterone into DHT. Saw palmetto and nettle root are often taken in capsule form.

Nettle is a beneficial reproductive tonic. Nettle root has shown cell proliferation inhibitory effect on prostate cancer cells via water-based extractions and alcohol-based extractions of the plant.[107] In other words, infusions as well as tinctures will work well for this purpose. I recommend combining nettle root tincture with daily nettle leaf infusions for full-spectrum action on the body. While nettle root works specifically with the prostate, helping manage DHT conversion as well as inhibiting the growth of prostate cancer cells, the nettle leaf infusion acts as a nutritive tonic, gentle diuretic, and vitality booster. Enjoy nettle root in tincture form or in capsules, while nettle leaf can be taken in the form of daily tonic infusions.

Dandelion leaf is a beneficial mineral-rich diuretic for better urinary flow. Dandelion leaf infusion also cleanses the body, provides nutrition, and supports the kidneys. The other healing part of dandelion, the root, promotes cancer cell apoptosis (which means the herb effectively "kills" cancer cells) and also increases the therapeutic benefits of chemotherapy treatment for prostate cancer.[108] I recommend using dandelion leaf as an infusion. It can be paired with nettle leaf along with other flavorful herbs like peppermint or ginger to spice up the taste. For the dandelion root, I recommend using it daily in the form of a tincture or in capsules.

Red clover supports prostate health. Epidemiological evidence shows that a high dietary intake of isoflavones, like the ones found abundantly in red clover, reduces the risk of prostate cancer and promotes general prostate health. Red clover slows or stops growth of prostate cancer through isoflavones-induced apoptosis in moderate-grade tumors. It is a promising remedy for prostate health in men with noncancerous, age-related prostate growth or enlargement.[109] Red clover blossoms are delicious in a tea infusion.

Cleavers is a beneficial diuretic and alterative herb. It is useful for urinary tract infections and prostatitis. It cools and shrinks the inflamed tissues of the urinary tract. Cleavers supports the kidneys and is an astringent tonic and anti-inflammatory. Paired with red clover, it works as a healing lymphatic tonic and gentle cleansing herbal ally for men and their sexual and reproductive health. Enjoy it as a tea or as freshly pressed cleavers juice in the warm season.

Sexually Transmitted Infections

Despite our best intentions, they happen. Sexually transmitted infections (STIs) are infectious diseases that are spread through sexual contact, be it oral, genital, or anal. STIs suck with a capital S, and they're very common. In fact, they are among the most common infectious diseases in the world today. There are more than twenty types of STIs, and they affect millions of people each year. Some of the most common include chlamydia, genital herpes, genital warts, and gonorrhea.

If you suspect you may have an STI, it's essential to get tested. With a diagnosis in hand, you can find herbal allies to assist you on your healing journey. Conventional treatment for STIs is a round of antibiotics. While this method is often effective, the concern around antibiotic resistance is growing—fast. Herbs may offer a safe alternative to antibiotics in some cases, and even when antibiotics are necessary, adding herbs to the antibiotic treatment may yield better results and lower the chance of recurrence when compared with using antibiotics alone.

> Many women find that a round of antibiotics leads to a vaginal yeast infection, which antifungal herbs like calendula can help remedy.

Herbs may not reverse STIs in every case, but they are effective strategies and treatment for symptom management and helping you find balance and ease in your sexual and reproductive life. Medicinal herbs contain naturally occurring phenolic and antioxidant compounds that show promise in the treatment of various types of STIs, be they parasitic diseases, microbial infections, or viruses. Herbs of special interest to folks dealing with STIs include natural broad-spectrum antimicrobials like garlic and Oregon grape or goldenseal, immunomodulators like reishi, immune stimulants like echinacea, and nervines like milky oats and lemon balm.

Chlamydia

Chlamydia infections affect the genitourinary system, or sexual organs and urinary tract. Early symptoms of chlamydia infection, like early symptoms of many STIs, may be misinterpreted as a urinary tract infection, with burning while peeing and pain in the lower abdomen. There can be redness, itching, and swelling in the genital area. It can cause a range of conditions, including cervicitis (inflammation of the cervix), urethritis (inflammation of the urethra), pelvic inflammatory disease, and infertility. Chlamydia infections may also be asymptomatic, which means it can be hard to tell whether you have it or not. That's why some people call chlamydia the "silent infection."

The conventional treatment for chlamydia is antibiotics. The first round of antibiotic treatment usually works well in curing chlamydia. But for folks who require more than one round of antibiotics, such as people who experience chronic chlamydia infection, the efficacy of treatment goes downhill fast. In many instances, *Chlamydia trachomatis* exhibits both antibiotic resistance and persistence. Antibiotic resistance in general is a huge concern when it comes to STIs. But antimicrobial herbs can help. And so do immune-modulating herbs.

Berberine is a natural compound found in the roots of the herbs Oregon grape, barberry, goldenseal, and coptis.[110] Research shows berberine kills bacteria by disrupting enzymes involved with making proteins and DNA/RNA. Berberine demonstrates activity against many harmful bacteria and shows promise in the treatment of vaginal chlamydia. You will find better results by using extracts made from the whole root rather than just the berberine because other phytochemicals present in the herb provide synergy and enhance the antibacterial effect of berberine. Enhance the immune system with reishi mushroom and add a soothing nervine like milky oats to support the nervous system while alkalizing the body.

Herpes

Herpes simplex virus 1 and 2 cause oral herpes and genital herpes, respectively. Oral herpes can lead to genital herpes following contact between a cold sore on the mouth and the genitals, such as via oral sex. As an infection for which conventional medicine has no cure, herpes sucks. But it doesn't have to be a death sentence for your sex life. The first outbreak tends to be the worst, with the most intense symptom levels in both severity and length. Herpes episodes can potentially reappear at any time, but herbal approaches to symptom management and lowering recurrence are effective and easy to implement.

St. John's wort is a beneficial antiviral that can be applied locally as an herbal oil or salve to both prevent and soothe sores. A blend of St. John's wort and lemon balm herbal oils, made by infusing plant material into an olive oil base, also delivers benefits to folks living with herpes.

Sitz baths are great too: soak the lower body and genital area in lemon balm tea to prevent and speed recovery from a herpes outbreak. Internally, use medicinal mushrooms such as reishi or cordyceps to support the immune system. Use milky oats as a tincture or herbal tea for a nervine tonic. It's well documented that a lowered immune system and stressed-out nervous system contribute to a higher likelihood of herpes outbreak recurrence.

If you follow good self-care habits and use beneficial herbs regularly, it's possible you'll never suffer from a herpes outbreak ever again after its first occurrence. Botanical therapies for oral and genital herpes involve the immune and nervous systems and consist of infection prevention and symptom relief. I've coached many herbal clients with herpes over the years, and this protocol has done wonders for them.

Propolis ointment applied to the skin may help both oral and genital lesions caused by herpes to heal faster. Propolis is a resin made by bees. A comparative multicenter study of ninety men and women with recurrent genital herpes (type 2) showed the beneficial effect of propolis on herpes sores.[III] Propolis ointment was compared with the conventional herpes and shingles medicine acyclovir (Zovirax) along with a placebo.

The ointments (propolis, acyclovir, and placebo) were all applied to the genital sores four times daily for thirty days. The propolis group was by far the fastest to heal. On day 10, twenty-four out of thirty folks in the propolis group had healed their genital sores, whereas only fourteen in the acyclovir and twelve in the placebo groups had healed their lesions.

Aside from applying propolis ointment, propolis tincture can also be taken internally for herpes relief. A study confirmed that conventional treatment for herpes sores is made more effective by the addition of propolis when used internally (ingested).[II2] The healing compounds in propolis show effect against herpes virus after only twenty-four hours of ingestion.

Lemon balm is an antiviral herb that is especially useful for preventing herpes outbreaks and providing relief for herpes sores. It is a gentle nervine and antidepressant herb. Lemon balm assists with the emotional aspect of STIs. Lemon balm is highly aromatic and tastes like a mix between mint and citronella. It extracts well in glycerin for a sweet-tasting remedy, or in alcohol for longer preservation.

St. John's wort is a nervine tonic and antiviral herb. It is soothing to frayed nerves and acts as an analgesic to alleviate pain and tension. It is a gentle antidepressant. Used topically as an herbal oil, St. John's wort is beneficial for soothing pain, itch, and burning of open herpes sores while helping accelerate wound healing.

Echinacea is an immune stimulant. Use it for short periods in acute cases and when infection is suspected. Echinacea delivers better results when it is paired with nutritive herbs and lymphatic tonics—herbs like nettle, reishi, and cleavers—to help with a strong immune system and the elimination of harmful invaders and toxins as well as the bacteria and viruses associated with STIs, including the herpes virus. The best time to use echinacea is when the first symptoms of a herpes outbreak appear. Take echinacea in the form of tincture or capsules when you feel that initial tingling or itching, and in the presence of other warning signs that a sore is imminent.

Reishi is a healing, adaptogenic mushroom and supreme immune tonic. Use reishi regularly and over long periods for best results, either in tincture form or capsules. Polysaccharides and triterpenoids from reishi show activity against herpes simplex virus and HIV.

Genital Warts

Genital warts are caused by a low-risk strain of human papillomavirus (HPV). The warts are skin growths in the groin, genital, or anal areas. They can take different sizes and shapes. Some are flat and others are bumpy. Herbs useful in the management of genital warts include immune-stimulating echinacea, adaptogenic astragalus, and andrographis (known as "Indian echinacea"). These herbal remedies are often taken in liquid tincture form.

In an open randomized trial of 261 patients with HPV-related anal warts who underwent surgery, an herbal blend containing echinacea and andrographis along with other herbs helped reduce the recurrence rate by a significant margin compared with those who did not use the herbs.[113] Astragalus can be safely taken over long periods. Use echinacea and andrographis when genital warts are present, and discontinue it when they go away. Medicinal mushrooms like reishi and turkey tail may be added to the protocol as well. For nervous system support, find the nervine herb with the highest affinity with you: it could be passionflower, milky oats, damiana, or other.

Gonorrhea

Gonorrhea is an STI caused by the bacteria *Neisseria gonorrhoeae*. The classic symptoms of gonorrhea include painful urination, urinary urgency, discharge from the vagina or penis, and soreness. The conventional treatment for gonorrhea is antibiotics. But what is happening now is that many bacteria and microbes such as *Neisseria gonorrhoeae* are becoming resistant to antibiotics due to overuse. Medicinal herbs have a lot to offer when it comes to managing the health risks associated with STIs and gonorrhea.

Goldenseal, which contains naturally occurring berberine, and garlic, which contains naturally occurring allicin, are two broad-spectrum antimicrobial herbs with a beneficial impact on gonorrhea infections. Take them in concentrated capsule form for best results. Turmeric, the golden spice that contains the naturally occurring active constituent curcumin, has also been studied for its potential against gonorrhea.[114] As with other STIs, nurturing the immune system with medicinal mushrooms and adaptogens is always indicated. Nervine herbs and nutritive herbs keep the body in a state of harmony that is better prepared to defend against bacterial infections.

UTIs and Urinary Health

Urinary tract infections (UTIs) can happen to anyone, but they commonly affect women, partly because their urethra is shorter (up to five times shorter than in males) and thus more prone to bacterial infection. Symptoms of UTIs include frequent urination, painful urination, a burning sensation while peeing, blood in the urine, pain in the lower abdomen, and the need to pee again despite having just urinated. A kidney infection is another type of UTI, which can become more serious if left untreated.

Symptoms of kidney infection include fever, chills, nausea or vomiting, and lower-back pain. Common symptoms of a UTI can mimic those of many STIs, so it's recommended to get tested in order to identify the cause with certainty and assess a better course of action and remedy. Because UTIs are caused by bacteria (most commonly *Escherichia coli*), they are conventionally treated with antibiotics. Many people who experience a UTI find that the infection returns following a round of antibiotics, which can set the stage for recurring and persistent UTIs. The urinary system responds well to herbal remedies.[115]

Diuretics like goldenrod, horsetail, and stinging nettle increase urine volume in both healthy people and people with urinary disorders, which helps in flushing out harmful bacteria. These herbs are often taken in the form of herbal infusions in the context of urinary infections. Horsetail, for instance, possesses therapeutic antibacterial activity and fights well against urinary tract pathogens like *E. coli, Klebsiella pneumoniae, Proteus mirabilis, Pseudomonas aeruginosa, Staphylococcus aureus, Staphylococcus saprophyticus,* and *Enterococcus faecalis.* Antibacterial phytochemical compounds found in horsetail include alkaloids, phytosterols, tannins, triterpenoids, and phenolic compounds like flavonoids.

Stinging nettle, on the other hand, exhibits antimicrobial activities against various Gram-positive and Gram-negative bacteria, such as *Bacillus subtilis, Lactobacillus plantarum, P. aeruginosa, E. coli, K. pneumoniae, S. aureus, and Staphylococcus epidermidis.*[116] Nettle leaf infusion in the treatment of UTI might be beneficial thanks to its diuretic action.

Antiseptic and antiadhesive herbs like uva-ursi deliver antimicrobial compounds, which may directly kill microbes or interfere with their adhesion to epithelial cells, thereby protecting against acute and chronic UTI. Uva-ursi, also known as bearberry or upland cranberry, is a useful herb for bladder infection as well. Uva-ursi leaves and herbal extracts made from them (often tinctures or tablets) have significant antibacterial activity, especially against the *E. coli* bacteria responsible for UTIs, and astringent activity due to uva-ursi's arbutin content and diuretic properties. In a double-blind study of fifty-seven women on the effect of uva-ursi on UTI recurrence compared with placebo, five of twenty-seven women had a recurrence in the placebo group while none of thirty women had a recurrence in the uva-ursi group after one year.[117]

Along with uva-ursi, the roots of Oregon grape and goldenseal are also beneficial to urinary health, thanks to the presence of naturally occurring berberine. Berberine is an important natural drug against many bacteria and combats infections by preventing the bacteria from adhering to the host cell, which suggests its potent role in treating UTI. The antibacterial activities of berberine against UTI directly interfere with the adhesion of *E. coli* to bladder cells and tissues. Finally, corn silk tea given to UTI patients significantly supported urinary health by reducing the presence of blood, pus, and crystals in the urine of folks with UTIs, without any side effects.

Overall, herbal strategies for urinary health target diuretic herbs like goldenrod, horsetail, and dandelion leaf for increased urine output and the flushing of bacteria. Urinary antiseptics such as goldenseal, coptis, uva-ursi, and corn silk are added to fight infection. Gentle demulcents like marshmallow root, slippery elm, and calendula soothe burning and inflammation, while alkalizing herbs such as milky oats, red clover, and nettle support wellness in the urinary system. The kidney tonics cleavers, nettle seed, or schisandra berry may be added, along with immuno-modulating herbs like reishi and astragalus when in the presence of recurrent UTIs.

Interstitial cystitis is a chronic urinary condition that may present like a chronic UTI. Along with following a similar protocol to the UTI herbal protocol, people with interstitial cystitis will strongly benefit from an emphasis on demulcent herbs (marshmallow root, slippery elm, calendula, aloe vera). Because interstitial cystitis often coexists with other inflammatory or immune conditions, it's recommended to add anti-inflammatory herbs like turmeric, antioxidant herbs like rosemary, and immune-modulating herbs or mushrooms like reishi.

Vaginal Microbiome

Just like the gut microbiome, the vagina possesses a fine and complex ecosystem in which beneficial flora crowd out pathogens. The vaginal flora keeps your vagina healthy and fends off harmful bacteria that may lead to infections like vaginitis. *Lactobacillus acidophilus* is one of the healthy bacteria that populate the vagina and keep it protected from imbalance and dysbiosis. *L. acidophilus* acts as an antimicrobial and acidifies the vagina by producing lactic acid. The vaginal flora protects against STIs and the development of pelvic inflammatory disease (PID).

Vaginal dysbiosis, or the disruption of the vaginal ecosystem and microbiome, is associated with vaginitis and can be traced to bacterial or fungal infection. Bacterial vaginosis (BV) is a common condition that leads to an unpleasant fishy odor, irritation, itching, and burning in the vagina. Yeast infections (often candida), or fungal vaginitis, cause similar symptoms to BV and may be episodic or recurrent and chronic. If you think you might have a vaginal infection, it's wise to get tested at a clinic to be sure. Overuse of antibiotics is a common cause of vaginitis, along with the use of scented intimate care products, perfumed soaps used on and around the vulva, and the use of conventional menstrual products.

When dealing with imbalances in the vaginal microbiome, herbs can help reestablish a balanced and whole ecosystem for better vaginal health. Some herbs that are best indicated for vaginal wellness in the context of infection and dysbiosis include calendula and goldenseal. Immune tonics like reishi, ashwagandha, schisandra, and holy basil support the body as a whole and prevent vaginal infections.

Finally, because stress is a huge factor in women's lives and affects the health of the vagina in both direct and indirect ways, nervine herbs like milky oats, passionflower, and damiana have a lot to offer and can be added to the vaginal health herbal protocol for best results.

Calendula is a potent antimicrobial herb. It fights off bacterial infection as well as fungal infection. A demulcent herb well suited to supporting the health and integrity of the vaginal mucosa, calendula can be used in an infused oil form, an infusion, a sitz bath, a yoni steam, and also in the form of tincture, capsule, and tea for internal use. In a 2018 study, a cream made with calendula extract was compared with metronidazole, a conventionally used antibiotic, on BV among women of reproductive age.[118] In this study, eighty women of reproductive age with diagnosed BV were randomly assigned to either the calendula group or the metronidazole group.

Both groups had a similar scale of symptoms, like vaginal burning and a fishy odor, but it was noted that the folks in the calendula group had the worst itching by far before the treatment started (22.5 percent versus 2.5 percent). Calendula extract or metronidazole vaginal cream (5 grams) was applied inside the vagina daily for a duration of one week. One week after the intervention, all women in both groups were free of symptoms, including vaginal itching and burning sensation, odor, and pain. In other words, calendula extract was as effective as the antibiotic for the treatment of BV, without any risks or side effects.

Goldenseal supports the vaginal microbiome. The naturally occurring compound berberine, which is found in goldenseal, coptis, barberry, and Oregon grape, fights against vaginal infections. A 2019 study on the effects of berberine on patients with bacterial vaginosis demonstrated that the cure rate of berberine is actually much higher than the cure rate associated with standard antibiotic treatment, with berberine ranking at a 92.8 percent cure rate compared with only a 75 to 86 percent cure rate with antibiotic treatment.[119] The dosage was a vaginal application of 0.3 grams of berberine applied daily for a duration of ten days per treatment for one month.

Goldenseal and other berberine-containing plants don't carry the side effects associated with antibiotics, and neither do they contribute to antibiotic resistance. For home use, goldenseal root or Oregon grape root (or other berberine-containing plant) can be infused in warm coconut oil over the stove for two to four hours. Strain and cool. Apply liberally around the vulva and inside the vagina until signs of infection go away.

7

Intimate Herbal Materia Medica

The following pages expand into herbal monographs for the herbs most commonly used within my intimate herbal practice. This is not an exhaustive list of all the herbs that could be considered sexual and reproductive tonics, hormone balancers, or otherwise beneficial to sexual health and fertility. Another herbalist may have chosen a different set of herbs altogether. But a good herbal, like a good wine, shows some character and personality, the imprint of terroir and culture. As such, these herbs make up my herbal practice centered on sexual and reproductive wellness and have become, over the last decade, indispensable allies in my tool kit. Once you add them to your herbal repertoire, I think you'll want to keep them around as well.

Ashwagandha

Withania somnifera

Ashwagandha belongs to the Solanaceae family. The part used is the root. Ashwagandha root has many medicinal properties relevant to sexual and reproductive health. It is an adaptogen, general tonic, anti-inflammatory, rejuvenator, nervous system tonic, aphrodisiac, mood-lifter, antianxiety, stress reliever, and thyroid support herb.

Ashwagandha is traditionally used as a general tonic and adaptogen. Today, ashwagandha is used to reverse chronic fatigue and sleep-wake disruptions caused by endocrine imbalance, shift work, jet lag, and symptoms of overwork or chronic stress. It is, like other adaptogens, a slow and steady builder and is best used over long periods. Ashwagandha root is taken as a tincture, in capsules, or in powder form when added to elixirs or energy balls. Whole dried.ashwagandha root can also be infused in wine for five to seven days. The taste of ashwagandha is reminiscent of soil and earth and blends beautifully with cacao, warm milk or milk alternative, and honey.

Ashwagandha replenishes fatigue and depletion while also bringing about more stable and uplifted energy levels. This might seem like a contradictory action, but a true tonic herb may first help relax and nourish you before it energizes you. On an intimate level, ashwagandha enhances stamina and fertility and reverses the effect of stress and burnout on libido and fertility. Its extract has been clinically shown to improve the quantity and health of sperm. Ashwagandha assists with hypothyroidism by balancing thyroid hormones, which in turns assists with mood, libido, weight regulation, and overall sexual and reproductive health. Biologically active chemical constituents in ashwagandha root include alkaloids, steroidal lactones (withanolides, withaferin), and saponins.

Modern science recognizes the beneficial impact of ashwagandha root on sexual and reproductive health and wellness. A prospective clinical study published in 2010 investigated the impact of ashwagandha on semen profile, oxidative biomarkers, and reproductive hormone levels in infertile men.[1] Dosage was 5 grams (roughly one teaspoon) of ashwagandha powder taken with milk daily for three months. The results of this study showed marked improvement in sperm concentration, sperm motility, and semen volume. The effects of ashwagandha also included reduced oxidative stress, increased serum testosterone and luteinizing hormone levels, and reduced levels of follicle-stimulating hormone and prolactin, all indicators of high semen quality.

While ashwagandha works in direct ways to enhance men's sexual health, women also benefit in more subtle ways—namely via stress and anxiety reduction. In a single-center, prospective, double-blind, randomized, placebo-controlled trial, participants with a history of chronic stress received a dosage of 300 milligrams of concentrated root extract twice daily for sixty days.[2] Results showed a significant reduction in scores on all the stress-assessment scales in the ashwagandha group, along with a substantial reduction in serum cortisol levels.

Native to India, Pakistan, Afghanistan, and Sri Lanka, ashwagandha is a staple herb of Ayurveda, the traditional medical system of India and Nepal, developed over three thousand years ago. It is known as a rasayana (restorative tonic) and is considered the "king of herbs," while shatavari is the queen.

The recommended dosage for ashwagandha root is 1–5 grams of powder per day, 2–5 milliliters of tincture per day, or 300 milligrams of concentrated root extract in capsule form twice daily.

Cacao

Theobroma cacao

Cacao belongs to the Malvaceae family. The part used is the seed. In an intimate herbal practice, cacao is enjoyed as a mood elevator, antidepressant, antioxidant, magnesium-rich heart tonic, and aphrodisiac herb.

Long revered as an energy food and aphrodisiac, cacao as a medicinal food is vastly different from what many of us have come to know as modern-day chocolate. Cacao has been used as a source of energy and stamina, for rituals and ceremonies, to open the heart, and to bring about a sense of well-being. Cacao is a traditional ally of lovers and is associated with love, sex, and sensuality.

Cacao is a powerhouse superfood rich in magnesium, antioxidants, and other mood-elevating and mind-boosting compounds. Among them is theobromine, a stimulating alkaloid that acts on the central nervous system and dilates blood vessels. Other high-functioning compounds in cacao include phenylethylamine, also known as the "love molecule," a mood-boosting substance that excites and arouses while providing a rush of energy, concentration, and alertness. Finally, cacao also contains anandamide, also called the "bliss chemical," which acts as a joy promoter;

reduces pain; regulates mood, appetite, and memory; and enhances cognitive flow.

Cacao is a stimulating nervine, which means it is best consumed in small intentional amounts. Avoid overreliance on cacao for a quick energy fix during conditions like intense stress, anxiety, and burnout. Cacao makes an ideal base for nutritionally potent medicinal herbs and herbal preparations. Enrich warm cacao drinks with maca and ashwagandha, for example, and transform dark chocolate barks into a vessel for other herbs, seaweed, and fungi.

Active constituents in cacao include antioxidants (epicatechin, gallic acid), flavanols, polyphenols, flavonoids and alkaloids, theobromine, phenethylamine, and anandamide. Cacao is rich in minerals such as iron, magnesium, phosphorus, manganese, zinc, and copper. Healthy saturated fats in cacao deliver fatty acids like oleic acid, palmitic acid, and stearic acid. The cacao seed can contain up to 40 to 60 percent solid fat.

Cacao delivers proven benefits for heart health, energy levels, and mood, all of which affect sexual and reproductive health in significant ways. A randomized, controlled, double-blind crossover trial in thirty healthy adults to investigate the effects of cacao flavanol on cognitive performance, anxiety, and mental fatigue showed that flavanol-rich cacao preparations significantly increased cognitive performance and reduced mental fatigue compared to the control group.[3]

Cacao lowers anxiety levels. A comprehensive assessment of the metabolic impact of cacao consumption in thirty subjects who consumed 40 grams of dark chocolate daily for a two-week period showed that cacao had significant anxiety-lowering effects in subjects who reported higher anxiety at the beginning of the study.[4] In these individuals, cacao consumption reduced urine cortisol and catecholamines while also normalizing other metabolic parameters associated with anxiety.

The protective effects of cacao on the cardiovascular system are widely studied. In a prospective study of 34,489 postmenopausal women free of cardiovascular disease, foods rich in flavonoids and other polyphenols abundant in cacao were associated with a decreased risk of coronary heart disease.[5] The Dutch Zutphen Study also highlights the protective effects of cacao intake.[6] After adjusting data to account for age, body mass index, lifestyle factors, diet, and caloric intake, the risk of cardiovascular disease for men who had the highest cacao intake was reduced by 50 percent compared with those who consumed the least amount of cacao. Cardiovascular disease is a common cause of erectile dysfunction and poor health outcomes overall.

Theobroma cacao, the cacao tree, has been around since ancient times. Cacao is native to the Amazon basin in South and Central America, where heirloom cacao trees still grow wild in the rain forests. Cacao trees live for up to a hundred years. Within each egg-shaped cacao pod there are twenty to forty cocoa beans, which are covered in a sweet white pulp. Cacao carries a long and rich history dating back to 1500 BCE. Named *xocolatl* by the Maya, the cacao bean was considered so valuable that it acted as currency in Mexico until the nineteenth century. The Olmecs of southern Mexico are believed to have been the first people to ferment, roast, and grind cacao beans for drinks and foods like porridge and gruel. The Maya, and later the Aztecs, drank cacao as a bitter and unsweetened, fermented beverage mixed with spices such as cayenne, vanilla, and cinnamon. Xocolatl and *cacahuatl* translate as "bitter water" in reference to their unsweetened drink and unprocessed, naturally bitter cacao bean.

Cacao was more than a food source, however. A sacred medicinal bean, cacao was involved in ceremonies and rituals, from marriages, burials, and offerings to the gods. It wasn't until the Spanish inquisition in the sixteenth century that cacao became popular outside of Mesoamerica. Hundreds of medicinal properties of cacao were cataloged in written resources of the time. The scientific name *Theobroma cacao* dates from the eighteenth century, when Swedish natural scientist Carl Linnaeus gave the cacao tree the name that translates as "food of the gods." Cacao trees were brought to West Africa in the 1800s. The hot and humid equatorial climate offered the perfect conditions for cacao cultivation. West Africa now produces over 70 percent of the world's cacao supply, with up to 90 percent of it grown on small family farms.

Cacao is taken in the form of dark chocolate, cacao powder, cacao nibs, and whole cacao beans. Take 15–35 grams of dark chocolate per day or 3–5 grams of cacao nibs, 3–4 whole cacao beans, or 3–5 grams of cacao powder once or twice a day.

Special Considerations Around Cacao

Who doesn't love cacao? The incredible popularity of cacao has turned the humble crop into a high-demand item. But the farming and production of cacao can be problematic when it is not done right. The human and environmental impacts are huge. From a human rights perspective, child labor, young migrant workers, and slavery are some top concerns when it comes to cacao production today. Roughly two-thirds of the world's cacao supply comes from the Ivory Coast and Ghana in West Africa, where an estimated two million children work as laborers on small cacao farms. There is no reliable or widespread certification for child labor–free cacao sourcing, so you need to do your research before buying any cacao and cacao products.

Many ethical "bean to bar" cacao companies are committed to fair trade, so there's no need to avoid the healing benefits of cacao altogether. Encourage ethical chocolatiers and support ethical sourcing. Other long-term solutions to eradicate child labor include worker cooperatives, higher prices for cacao that would support living wages, and wider poverty alleviation. As a solution, cacao farmers are trying to sell their cacao themselves without the overbearing middlemen who buy from small farmers to resell on the market at a high markup that the farmers and workers never benefit from. Environmentally speaking, unsustainable cacao farming has proved to be damaging to the earth as well.

Monocrops, hybrids, pesticide and chemical fertilizer use, soil depletion, and loss of biodiversity are some of the common issues associated with contemporary cacao farms. Solutions include organic farming, regenerative farming practices, and farm diversification.

There are three main varieties of cacao: Forastero, Criollo, and Trinitario. More recently, Arriba Nacional has been added to the list of cacao bean varieties. Forastero is the most common cacao crop, accounting for about 90 percent of the cacao trees cultivated today. Forastero is hardy, high-yield, and disease-resistant, and is popular in West African cacao plantations. Criollo, Trinitario, and Arriba Nacional make up about 10 percent of the cacao plantings worldwide: Criollo and Arriba Nacional 3 percent, and Trinitario 7 percent. These cacao families are grown in Peru, Venezuela, Ecuador, and Mexico, among other places. Many farmers, some of them indigenous, reclaim their heritage with heirloom cacao farming today in a way that benefits both people and the earth. Some cacao farmers and farmer co-ops continue to grow and harvest cacao as a family tradition and cultural practice.

Calendula

Calendula officinalis

Calendula belongs in the Asteraceae family. The part used for medicinal purposes is the flower. Calendula flower has anti-inflammatory, antibacterial, antispasmodic, lymphatic, and emmenagogue properties that are useful in the context of herbalism for sexual and reproductive health.

Calendula is a classic herb of the modern pharmacopeia and often one of the first medicinal herbs folks will get introduced to when they start their journey with herbalism. It's a must-have all-around remedy with a wide variety of uses. For intimate herbalism, calendula is a beneficial antimicrobial herb useful in the context of vaginitis, urinary tract infections, and as a soothing salve over herpes sores, among others. Calendula can be used internally as a tincture or infusion and can be used externally as an oil or salve.

When consumed as a tea or tincture, calendula acts as a potent lymphatic tonic that moves the lymph and supports the immune system, especially in the context of breast cysts or other breast conditions like breast cancer. Calendula oil or salve has a strong affinity with the mucosa of the genitals, be it the tip of the penis, inside the vagina and anus, and other tender tissues that can get inflamed or irritated and need soothing. It makes a superb herbal lubricant, either in oil for use without condoms, or infused in vegetable glycerin for use with condoms (which are incompatible with oil). Active constituents in calendula flower include flavonoids, polysaccharides, volatile oil, and terpenes.

The effect of calendula extract in treating bacterial vaginosis was tested in a double-blind, randomized, controlled trial group of eighty women of reproductive age.[7] Half the group was treated with an alcohol-based extract of calendula, and the other half was treated with metronidazole. After one week, all women reported having no symptoms of bacterial vaginosis, and calendula was deemed to be a safe and effective treatment without the side effects of synthetic drugs.

A randomized controlled trial on the effect of calendula on the treatment of vaginal candidiasis and sexual function was examined against the treatment with clotrimazole.[8] A group of 150 women of reproductive age were treated with either calendula or clotrimazole vaginal cream (5 milligrams) every night for seven nights. Treatment with calendula cream took longer to become effective, but had a greater long-term effect on symptoms of candidiasis than clotrimazole. Both treatments effectively improved sexual function.

There is some evidence for the use of calendula in the prevention and treatment of STIs. While a lower amount of *Lactobacillus acidophilus* in the vaginal ecosystem is associated with a higher risk of infection, calendula extract applied over the genitals provides a healthier vaginal ecosystem in which infection cannot survive.[9] In this particular example, calendula is combined with herbal extracts of ginger, clove, green tea, and garlic.

Calendula is believed to have been one of the first cultivated flowers, having originated in Egypt and brought to Britain by the Romans. Calendula has been enjoyed by humans for centuries for its bright and cheerful disposition in the garden and as an edible and useful medicine plant.

The recommended dosage for calendula is 1–4 grams of flower (fresh: use more; dried: use less) infused in water up to three times daily, or 1–2 milliliters of tincture three times daily. As an herbal oil or salve, apply over the desired area as needed.

Cleavers

Galium aparine

Cleavers belongs in the Rubiaceae family. The parts used in intimate herbalism are the flowers, leaves, and stems—in other words, the whole aerial

parts. Cleavers possesses many beneficial properties for sexual and reproductive wellness. It is a diuretic, alterative, anti-inflammatory, tonic, and
astringent herb.

Cleavers is a cleansing herb and has traditionally been used to awaken the
body in the springtime after a long winter. Cleavers has an affinity for the lymphatic system and moves stagnation through the body. The lymphatic system
is cleansed by using cleavers as it moves lymph and toxins through the body.
This is particularly useful for reawakening the immune system in the spring.

Cleavers is a diuretic and has demulcent properties that are soothing
to the kidneys and the urinary system, and the herb is especially useful in
the treatment of urinary tract infections (UTIs). It is a valuable remedy for
cystitis, BPH, prostatitis, chronic UTIs, and interstitial cystitis. Cleavers is
cooling and reduces inflammation throughout the urinary tissues, including the bladder and urethra and genitourinary system overall.

Active constituents in cleavers include phenols, tannins, alkaloids,
anthraquinones, coumarins, iridoids, asperuloside, alkanes, flavonoids,
and saponins. Cleavers has been one of the herbs used in formulations by
naturopaths for the treatment of acute UTIs.[10] One case study reported that
a woman with recurring UTIs had no recurrence of urinary tract infection
for one year while using an herbal formulation that contained cleavers for
its demulcent and lymph-stimulating properties.

A 2016 study on the effect of cleavers against breast cancer cells showed
that cleavers is a beneficial and valid remedy to slow the spread of breast
cancer.[11] Within only seventy-two hours after use, cleavers extract exerts
toxicity against breast cancer cell lines while remaining safe to normal
healthy breast tissue.

Cleavers is one of those underappreciated edible and medicinal plants
that thrive in human-generated anthropogenic habitats like garden beds,
sidewalk cracks, trailheads, and just about anywhere the soil has been disrupted. Herbs like cleavers, along with dandelion, burdock, and St. John's
wort, have been categorized as weeds or invasives, but this limited view
overlooks their therapeutic actions.

The same qualities that make certain plants "invasive" also allow them
to thrive in stressful, climatically unstable environments. They rely on

active constituents that, once consumed by humans in the form of herbal remedies, offer us an advantage in the context of stressful and unstable environments as well. In this era of rapidly changing ecosystems and concern over endangered and overharvested species, "weeds" like cleavers show up as abundant sources of resilient, adaptable, energy-efficient, and sustainable food and medicine for humans, animals, and the earth.

Recommended dosage for cleavers is 2–4 grams herb infused in water as an infusion up to three times daily, or 2–4 milliliters of liquid extract (tincture) three times daily. Cleavers can also be applied topically as an herbal oil or salve, as needed.

Damiana
Turnera aphrodisiaca or *Turnera diffusa*

Damiana belongs in the Turneraceae family. The part used for therapeutic purposes is the leaf. Damiana is a nervous system tonic, a sexual tonic, and an antidepressant and aphrodisiac herb.

It has a long history of use as a potent sexual tonic as well as an uplifting, antidepressant herbal ally. As a nervine herb, damiana particularly benefits those who suffer from chronic stress, tension, and low moods. Damiana pairs well with nervine trophorestorative milky oats, along with other popular tonics like ashwagandha and rosemary. Damiana extracts well into liqueur, which explains its popularity as a luscious, mood-altering drink. The taste of damiana alcoholic extract is minty, woody, floral, slightly bitter, and undeniably herbal. It is rumored that the original margaritas were made with damiana liqueur. Damiana is also enjoyed as part of an herbal smoke blend, as well as in herbal baths and soaks.

Active constituents in damiana include flavonoids, volatile oil, resin, and damianin. A placebo-controlled study of 108 women aged twenty-two to seventy-three with low libido researched the effect of a damiana and ginkgo vitamin and mineral supplement.[12] The daily serving of herbs in the supplement included 2,700 milligrams of a blend of L-arginine, Korean ginseng, *Ginkgo biloba,* and damiana leaf. The women taking the supplement reported a 72 percent increase in sexual desire and a 68 percent increase in satisfaction with overall sex life compared with the placebo group after only four weeks of treatment with the damiana blend.

An animal study showed that damiana extract is as effective as Valium in reducing anxiety, without the risks and side effects associated with diazepam and other benzodiazepines.[13] This confirms the long history of use of damiana as a potent antidepressant and antianxiety ally in folk medicine.

Damiana is native to Texas, New Mexico, Baja California, and other parts of Mexico. Damiana use has been traced back to the Guaycura indigenous people who occupied Baja California's Cedros Island as early as 9,000 to 10,000 years ago. Damiana was later enjoyed by the Aztecs and Maya.

The recommended dosage for damiana is 2–4 milliliters of tincture up to three times per day. As an infusion, use 1 teaspoon of dried herb per cup of boiling water, and steep for ten to fifteen minutes. Drink up to three cups per day. Herbal baths are another wonderful way to enjoy damiana medicine.

Dandelion

Taraxacum officinale

Dandelion belongs in the Asteraceae family. Every part of the dandelion is medicinal. In an intimate herbal practice, the parts used are the root and the leaf. Dandelion has depurative, diuretic, cholagogue, bitter, tonic, and liver-cleansing properties.

In traditional plant medicine, dandelion root is one of the most detoxifying herbs and works primarily on the liver and gallbladder to release waste products. By supporting the liver, excessive estrogens and toxins can be deactivated. Cleansing the liver is important because it is the site of hormone processing. If the liver is cleansed, hormones are processed quickly and efficiently, avoiding buildups or imbalances in the body. This can then lead to a regulation of hormone cycling in the body and support overall sexual and reproductive health. The root of dandelion is used to increase secretions in the stomach, liver, and pancreas. This action encourages liver detoxification. Dandelion also cleanses through its diuretic action on the kidneys.

Dandelion is useful in the context of enlarged prostate to enhance urinary output, and also supports elimination of urine during urinary tract infections. Premenstrually and during the luteal phase of the ovarian cycle, dandelion root can be used for its diuretic properties, which can help with fluid retention. Many women report gaining up to seven pounds during the luteal phase, most of it as fluid, which dandelion extract eliminates.

In Traditional Chinese Medicine, dandelion is used to expel heat and fire and dispel heat in the lower burner.[14] Dandelions are a cold plant from an energetics standpoint and so help to treat individuals with an excess of heat in the body. If you've ever had a urinary tract infection and its associated "burning pee," a cooling herb will no doubt sound really good right now!

In Traditional Chinese Medicine the liver is referred to as the body's general and is thought to play a role in balancing emotions. Fertility-wise, folks undergoing IVF or preparing for a treatment may seek dandelion extract to help with hormone regulation in pursuit of successful in vitro fertilization treatments. Along with dandelion root, dandelion leaf extract acts as a superior kidney tonic. In Traditional Chinese Medicine, kidney essence governs birth, vitality, and reproduction. It provides direction, energy, and substance to the reproductive system.[15]

Active constituents in dandelion include sesquiterpene lactones, triterpene steroids, phenolic acids, and polysaccharides. Dandelion has been used traditionally for centuries, and some scientific studies have been done on its efficacy. A 2007 animal study on reproductive hormone regulation examined whether the use of dandelion extract would upregulate estrogen receptors, progesterone receptors, and follicle-stimulating hormone receptors.[16] Higher mRNA expression of estrogen receptors, higher estrogen and progesterone receptors in the uterus, and higher follicle-stimulating hormone receptors were found in the subjects with the dandelion extract after a treatment period of only six weeks.

Another recent study looked at the use of dandelion extract on ovarian granulosa cells and found that granulosa cell viability increased with increasing concentrations of dandelion extract.[17] This study concluded that dandelion extract, through steroid hormone synthesis, can cause proliferation of granulosa cells and upregulation of granulosa cell expression, which increases ovarian function overall. This is of specific interest to folks working with fertility treatments like IVF because this regulating action on the hormones could be linked to the success of in vitro fertilization in patients with low ovarian function.

Dandelion has nearly global distribution on earth and its leaves and roots have been used as a nutrient-dense food by many cultures across the globe. North American indigenous peoples use dandelion as a cleanser for the urinary tract and the digestive system. The Native American Ethnobotany Database returns seventy-one matches of dandelion by different North American indigenous groups.[18] Uses are varied and include use as a tonic, for swollen testicles and menstrual cramps, and to increase lactation.

Recommended dosage for dandelion in the form of infusion is 4–10 grams in water up to three times per day. In tincture form, take 2–5 milliliters up to three times per day.

Ginger

Zingiber officinale

Ginger belongs in the Zingiberaceae family. The part used is the root (rhizome). Ginger has many beneficial properties for sexual and reproductive health. It is a digestive, warming, circulatory tonic, antispasmodic, anti-inflammatory, and highly aromatic herb.

Ginger is a warming aromatic spice traditionally used to support digestion, enhance circulation, and to relieve pain and nausea associated with the menstrual cycle and endometriosis. It can be enjoyed in numerous ways: ginger is delicious added to foods, whether fresh or dried as powder. Ginger soda, ginger syrup, ginger kombucha, ginger tincture in alcohol or glycerin, and other liquid concoctions are delicious and therapeutic. Ginger candies as well as ginger capsules may be used as well.

Active constituents in ginger include bioactive volatile oils responsible for its strong aroma. Ginger also delivers oleoresins such as gingerols, phenols, flavonoids, vitamin C, vitamin E, beta-carotene, lutein, lycopene, quercetin, genistein, tannins, manganese, copper, selenium, and zinc.

One of the most researched benefits of ginger in relation to sexual and reproductive health—aside from its effect on pregnancy-related morning sickness—is in the relief of dysmenorrhea (painful periods). A study published in 2009 reported that ginger capsules were as effective as ibuprofen in relieving pain associated with dysmenorrhea.[19] The double-blind comparative clinical trial studied 150 women with dysmenorrhea. The dosage used was 250 milligrams of ginger rhizome powder in capsule form, four times a day for three days from the start of their menstrual period. Ginger can also be used in the context of endometriosis for the same pain-relieving and antispasmodic action. Ginger pairs well with valerian root and turmeric root for that purpose.

Another interesting avenue for the therapeutic use of ginger is in its fertility-supporting benefits for infertile men. A 2012 study showed that ginger supplementation over a three-month period increased sperm count (16.2 percent), motility (47.3 percent), viability (40.7 percent), normal morphology (18.4 percent), and ejaculate volume (36.1 percent).[20] There were significant increases in serum FSH, LH, and testosterone levels after the ginger treatment compared with before treatment. The study participants were seventy-five infertile men ranging in age from nineteen to forty. The dosage was not specified. Standard dosage for ginger averages 1–3 grams per day.

Ginger first appeared in the southern parts of ancient China. From there, it spread to India, the Maluku Islands (an archipelago in eastern Indonesia), the rest of Asia, and West Africa. Ginger shares a plant family with its cousins cardamom and turmeric. It was an important player in the spice trade that endured through the Middle Ages and was exported from India to the Roman Empire, where it was especially valued for its medicinal properties, over two thousand years ago.

The recommended dosage for ginger is 1–3 milliliters of tincture up to four times per day. As an infusion, take 1 teaspoon of ginger per cup of water. In powder form, enjoy 1–5 grams per day. In capsules, take 550 milligrams up to four times per day, or a 1,000-milligram capsule twice daily. Enjoy ginger fresh, dried, pickled, candied, crystalized, powdered, infused, or in other forms.

Hawthorn

Crataegus spp.

Hawthorn belongs in the Rosaceae family. The parts commonly used within intimate herbalism are the leaves, flowers, and berries. Hawthorn is a heart tonic with antioxidant and hypotensive properties.

In China and Europe, hawthorn has a long documented history of use in herbal medicine. Hawthorn is traditionally used as a heart tonic. Based on its connection to the heart, hawthorn is also used in energy medicine and as a flower essence for expanding the emotional heart. Hawthorn can be used to encourage self-love and self-acceptance. Hawthorn may be useful in opening the heart to love and connection from others and the self.

Active constituents in hawthorn include amines, flavonoids, tannins, glycosides, and saponins. A review of the use of hawthorn in the treatment of cardiovascular disease found the plant to be potentially safe and effective for both cardiovascular disease and ischemic heart disease.[21] Hawthorn holds many benefits for men experiencing erectile dysfunction, which may be commonly associated with low cardiovascular function.

Hawthorn represents fertility and it is commonly used as a part of Beltane celebration on May 1. Hawthorn is also symbolic of the heart in Christianity due to its ability to open the heart to love. When my husband and I first started dating, he had a dream one night that I harvested and offered him hawthorn berries. He took it as a sign that he was ready to open his heart to me.

The recommended dosage for hawthorn is 0.3–1.0 grams of the herb as an infusion three times daily, or 1–2 milliliters of tincture up to three times daily.

Maca

Lepidium meyenii

Maca belongs to the Brassicaceae family. The part used is the root. Maca has therapeutic properties as an adaptogen, aphrodisiac, nutritive, and hormone-balancing herb.

Maca grows in the Peruvian mountains and meets its specific growing needs in the mineral-rich volcanic soil of the harsh high-altitude Andes. It is a cruciferous root vegetable that belongs to the same family as cabbage, radish, and turnip. It is high in iron and calcium and contains copper, zinc, and potassium. It is believed that maca root was consumed by the Incas to provide strength and nourishment during times of famine.

Often enjoyed today in the form of powder and mixed into bliss balls or smoothie blends, dried maca root powder has a strong affinity with fertility. The high nutrient content of maca supports healthy sexual response, increases fertility, and deeply nourishes the body. As an adaptogen, maca increases body resilience and builds a better capacity to engage in daily tasks and demands. Maca works on the endocrine level and supports hormonal balance. It should come as no surprise that with all these juicy benefits, maca shows up as a trusted aphrodisiac, helping you reconnect to your sensual nature. Maca is beneficial during menopause. With a sweet taste reminiscent of malty caramel, maca root powder blends delightfully with cacao for a tasty superfood drink.

Active constituents in maca root include protein, essential amino acids, iron, calcium, carbohydrates, lipids, fiber, and linoleic, palmitic, and oleic acids. The secondary metabolites macaridine, macaene, macamides, and maca alkaloids are only found in this plant. Macaenes are unsaturated fatty acids. Other compounds include sterols as beta-sitosterol, campesterol, and stigmasterol.

Maca's effects on male and female reproductive capacity have been examined in vivo and in human studies. Clinical trials show the efficacy of maca on sexual dysfunctions as well as for increasing sperm quality. In a study in nine healthy men who had received maca for four months, results showed an increase in seminal volume, sperm count, and sperm motility.[22]

A 2002 randomized, double-blind, placebo-controlled study of men treated with maca sought to examine the effect on sexual desire, mood, and serum testosterone levels.[23] The men, aged between twenty-one and fifty-six, were treated with maca at a dosage of 1,500 milligrams, 3,000 milligrams, or a placebo. Measures of sexual desire, depression, and anxiety were recorded at four, eight, and twelve weeks. Male sexual desire increased in the groups undergoing treatment using maca at eight and twelve weeks, regardless of depression and anxiety scores.

In 2015, a twelve-week, double-blind, placebo-controlled trial of maca root in forty-five women ages eighteen to sixty-five with antidepressant-induced sexual dysfunction demonstrated the safe and effective aphrodisiac properties of maca.[24] The dosage was 3 grams of maca root powder per day. In a previous trial, women consuming this daily dose had described greater sexual activity and more enjoyable sexual experiences. It is worth noting that the beneficial effects of maca on sexual, arousal, and orgasmic function are multiplied in postmenopausal women.

Maca has been cultivated in the Peruvian central Andes and was domesticated for cultivation some 1,300 to 2,000 years ago.[25] The first written description about maca was published in 1553. The fertility-promoting benefits of maca were noted in written records as early as 1653. Traditionally, maca root is dried after harvesting and is stored in the same way as other root vegetables like potatoes and turnips. Before eating, the dried roots are boiled into a soft porridge. These days, maca root is most commonly enjoyed in dried powder form and added to drinks, smoothies, and cacao.

The recommended dosage for maca is 1–5 grams of powder up to twice a day. Take 1–3 milliliters of tincture up to twice per day, or maca capsules at a dosage of 1,000–3,000 milligrams up to twice per day.

Mushrooms

Medicinal mushrooms belong to the fungal community. They are potent adaptogens, immunomodulators, and tonics. Important constituents in medicinal mushrooms include polysaccharides like beta-D-glucans, polysaccharopeptides (PSP), polysaccharide proteins, triterpenes, lipids, and phenols.

Taken daily, medicinal mushrooms bring vitality, energy, and strong immunity and enhance sexual wellness. They possess potent anticancer effects that protect against many cancers, including breast cancer, ovarian cancer, and prostate cancer. They also offer liver-protective benefits that protect against liver dysfunction and hormonal imbalances.

Mushrooms and fungi used for medicinal purposes in the context of intimate herbalism include reishi *(Ganoderma)*, cordyceps *(Cordyceps sinensis)*, lion's mane *(Hericium erinaceus)*, turkey tail *(Trametes versicolor)*, maitake *(Grifola frondosa)*, and shiitake *(Lentinula edodes)*, among others. They are commonly consumed in the form of decoctions, tinctures, capsules, and powders.

Cordyceps mushroom offers interesting benefits for fertility and reproductive function.[26] Studies conducted in the 1980s showed that a cordyceps supplement was effective in increasing sperm count by 33 percent, decreasing sperm malformations by 29 percent, and increasing sperm survival rate by 79 percent in twenty-two male participants over a period of only eight weeks of treatment. Another study reported a 300 percent improvement in sperm count in infertile men following treatment with cordyceps mushroom. Finally, intake of cordyceps is strongly associated with a sharp increase in libido.

Reishi has been studied for its protective effect against HIV and AIDS due to its antiviral action. In the same way, reishi supplementation is considered useful in the context of sexually transmitted infections like herpes.[27]

The recommended dosage for medicinal mushrooms is 2–5 milliliters of tincture up to four times daily. In powder form, use 5 grams up to three times daily. In capsules, take the equivalent of two 500-milligram capsules up to three times daily. Mushroom powders can be added to coffee, tea, smoothies, or elixirs. Culinary mushrooms like shiitake, oyster mushroom, and other edible mushrooms can also be enjoyed for their healing benefits.

Nettle

Urtica dioica

Nettle belongs to the Urticaceae family. The parts used in intimate herbalism are the leaf, seed, and root. Nettle leaf is the portion of the plant that is particularly rich in nutrients. Nettle root contains diuretic properties, for which it is used in the treatment of disorders associated with enlarged prostate. Nettle seed is considered a functional food. It contains a plethora of healthful vitamins and minerals and is a kidney trophorestorative. Nettle has nutritive and tonic properties. It is a nutrient-rich, adaptogen-like functional food.

It is rich in bioavailable vitamins, minerals, chlorophyll, sterols, flavonoids, and other nutrients. Many herbalists consider nettle to act as an adaptogen, increasing resilience of body and mind and nurturing every organ and body system in both direct or indirect ways.

Nettle leaf is not a reproductive system–specific or hormonal herb–specific ally but is a nutritive tonic rich in vitamins and minerals (and an especially iron-rich tonic). Traditionally, nettle infusion aids with the low energy associated with heavy menstruation. The leaves contain chlorophyll, vitamins A, D, C, K, and B complex, proteins, phosphorus, iron, sulfur, and magnesium. The seeds contain fatty acids, sterols, and tocopherols.

In a 2011 randomized, double-blind, placebo-controlled study of participants with benign prostatic syndrome (BPS), participants using stinging nettle root extract after one year had fewer complications due to the disease, including lower incidence of urinary tract infections.[28]

Nettle is found nearly worldwide as a common weed and is thought of as a nuisance plant by farmers working the land, who brush their hands or legs inadvertently over the weedy sprawling plants and experience an instant, but temporary, burning pain on the skin. Historically, nettle has been a celebrated medicinal herb and was heartily recommended by the German abbess and healer Hildegard von Bingen. In the Middle Ages in Europe, before the 1516 Bavarian purity law that decreed only barley, hops, and water were allowed in beer-making, nettle beer was a popular drink.

Much of the world's nettle production today is not cultivated but rather still a foraged harvest, coming from Slavic countries where the sustainable wild foraging traditions have been kept alive. The top exporters of quality wild nettles are Albania, Bosnia and Herzegovina, Bulgaria, and Hungary, where they have implemented the organic wild-crop harvesting practice standard for certified-organic wild-collected nettle.

According to Gayle Engels at the American Botanical Council and botanical supply-chain expert and researcher Josef Brinckmann, some of these organic wild-harvested nettle operations have also adopted the Fair-Wild standard, which includes criteria not only for ecological sustainability but also for economic and social sustainability for the harvesters and their communities.[29]

The recommended dosage for nettle is 2–4 grams of herb per cup of water as an infusion taken three times daily. In tincture form, take 2–6 milliliters three times daily. Nettle can be consumed as food. Nettle leaf may be used similarly to spinach, and nettle seeds similarly to sesame seeds.

Oats

Avena sativa

Oats belong in the Poaceae family. The parts used in the context of sexual and reproductive wellness are the milky oat seed and the whole aerial parts (also called oat straw). Oats are a nervine, a nervous system trophorestorative, and a nutritive, antioxidant, antidepressant, and anxiolytic herb. Oats are a cardiac tonic and blend well with hawthorn for this use.

As a traditional nervous system trophorestorative and a potent nutritive herb, oats are commonly used in cases of high anxiety, depression, and fatigue. Taken over long periods, milky oats boost stamina and strength. Milky oats are recommended in cases of nervous exhaustion, depression, insomnia, and burnout. A quintessential herbal ally for our busy hectic times, oats strengthen a weakened nervous system and restore balance on a physical, spiritual, and emotional level. For anyone who struggles with sexual and reproductive wellness, fertility, and cycles, milky oats offer therapeutic benefits and myriad healing and balancing actions.

Milky oats can be considered a sexual appetite booster. As a nourishing herb, it assists with blood flow and heart health, especially when paired with hawthorn. Milky oats are a gently stimulating nervine, nourishing and calming the nerves while increasing sensitivity to your surroundings and your ability to be fully present in the moment.

Milky Oats or Oat Straw?

Medicinal oats can be consumed as oat straw or as milky oats. Oat straw is the aerial part of the plant and includes the stem and leaf. It's most often used as a nutritive tonic because of its high vitamin and mineral content, perfect for nourishing and soothing the worn-out, exhausted, and depleted person. Milky oats, on the other hand, are the oat seeds harvested during the milky latex stage of development, before they have fully ripened. Oat tops in that milky stage possess a strong medicinal tonic and restorative action on the nervous system. Milky oats can be tinctured fresh in alcohol right after harvest or dried whole.

Milky oat seed is a great source of healing nutrients, including vitamin E in the form of tocopherols and tocotrienols, B vitamins, iron, manganese, zinc, calcium, silicon, and selenium, along with choline and phosphatidyl-choline. Active constituents in milky oats include triterpenoid saponins; protein (avenins, gluten); polyphenols; monosaccharides and oligosaccharides; nutrients such as iron, manganese, zinc, and calcium; and glycosyl flavones.

A 2020 study on the effects of green oat extract on mood and stress regulation adopted a dose-ranging, double-blind, randomized parallel groups design in which 132 healthy people aged thirty-five to sixty-five received either 430 milligrams, 860 milligrams, or 1,290 milligrams green oat extract or placebo for twenty-nine days. The study demonstrated that milky oats regulate the stress response, effectively lowering insomnia, anxiety, and other stress responses that are harmful to sexual and reproductive health.[30]

Recent studies validate the traditional use of oats as an aphrodisiac, with beneficial impact in the context of low libido, erectile dysfunction, and stress.[31] A 2018 study showed that a triple combination of oats, *Tribulus*, and ginseng together was particularly efficient for improving male sexual dysfunction.[32]

From an ethnobotanical perspective, oats make a great addition to the home garden. According to Latina *mamita*, clinical herbalist, and community organizer Lara Pacheco, oats offer benefits to both the garden, the gardener, people, and soil.[33] The immature seed pod, in its milky stage, yields succulent milky juice for a potent nervous system medicine. The stems and leaves, on the other hand, can be harvested and dried for oat straw, which makes a nourishing tea rich in vitamins and minerals. And the plant itself, along with its roots, make an excellent cover crop or green manure, which provides therapy for the soil.

Lara teaches that, in the garden, milky oats can act as a cover crop to protect, rebuild, and give rest to the cultivated earth by stabilizing the soil and bioaccumulating calcium and magnesium. Lara notes that the way we engage with the soil in our capitalist system is similar to the way we marginalize and mistreat people. In our industrial agricultural system, soil is treated as a simple inorganic one-dimensional means of production, and as such, it is put under a great deal of stress in order to constantly maximize high yields of the same crop, year after year, without rest or replenishment.

In the same way, capitalist culture treats people as simple means of production and consumption. In both the case of soil and people, this system denies the rich diversity and totality of existence, of which rejuvenation and nourishment are an integral, holistic part. In the same way that oats can bring nourishment to the tired and overworked soil, so it acts on the tired overworked nervous system, and in doing so, acts as a supreme ally for sexual and reproductive health and wellness, especially when paired with a nutritive tonic like nettle.

The recommended dosage for oats medicine is 1 tablespoon of milky oats or oat straw infused in one cup of water; drink as needed. Take 1–5 milliliters of tincture daily.

Red Clover

Trifolium pratense

Red clover belongs to the Fabaceae family. The part used therapeutically is the flower. Red clover is a nutritive and alterative herb that provides immune support and endocrine support.

Traditionally, red clover has been used in herbal medicine for the treatment of menopause and lymphatic disorders. Due to its high nutrient content, red clover may be used in preparation for pregnancy. Red clover has strong action as a blood cleanser and has traditionally been used for this purpose. The flavonoids in red clover are phytoestrogens that mimic estrogen in the body, and the plant has a long history of use in women's health. Particularly, estrogen is commonly used for the treatment of menstrual and menopausal symptoms.

Red clover also promotes the movement of lymph through the lymphatic tissues. The breasts contain lymphatic tissue that can become stagnant, decreasing the body's immune defense system. Using red clover to increase the movement of lymphatic fluid, especially through larger sites such as the breasts, helps to remove toxins from the body as well as ensure that immune cells are functioning properly. Stagnation of the lymph can lead to various other infections and conditions when the body is not able to effectively eliminate them and protect itself, which red clover helps mediate.

Active constituents in red clover include isoflavones, carbohydrates, coumarins, flavonoids, saponins, and salicylic acid. A meta-analysis of the literature found that peri- and postmenopausal women had significantly fewer hot flashes when taking red clover.[34] A dosage of 80 milligrams of red clover showed a significant decrease in the occurrence of hot flashes. A similar study found that at three to four months, there was a significant difference between hot flashes in the control group and the red clover treatment group.[35] Note that this difference was not found at twelve months, which suggests that short-term use of red clover may be the wisest approach when used for this condition.

Red clover originated in Europe, western Asia, and northwest Africa and has since developed a global distribution. Red clover is also reported to have been a sacred plant to the Romans and Greeks, who associated the plant with their triple goddesses.

The recommended dosage for red clover is 4 grams of dried flower per cup of water up to three times daily. In tincture form, take 1–2 milliliters up to three times daily.

Red Raspberry Leaf

Rubus idaeus

Red raspberry leaf belongs in the Rosaceae family. The part used therapeutically is the leaf. Red raspberry leaf offers beneficial properties as a nutritive tonic, mineral builder, uterine tonic, and astringent herb.

Traditionally, it is used as a uterine tonic. Use it as an herbal tea and pair with nettle leaf for a nutritive tonic action. Red raspberry leaf fortifies and provides the body with highly absorbable vitamins C, E, A, and B complex as well as minerals like iron, magnesium, calcium, and potassium. Like nettle, red raspberry leaf is another humble local "weed" that fits into a carbon-zero bioregional approach to herbal medicine for those who live in the northern hemisphere—easy to grow yourself and easier still to forage wild. And like nettle, red raspberry leaf acts as a deeply restorative nutritive tonic rich in highly bioavailable vitamins and minerals.

Red raspberry leaf allies with the uterus from the early years all through menopause. Like nettle, red raspberry leaf is thoroughly enjoyed in the form of a tasty infusion—pair with nettle, oat tops, ginger, and hibiscus for a hot-pink and lavish sip.

Herbalist Richard Whelan believes that red raspberry leaf blends well with lady's mantle for a weakened uterus, with shepherd's purse for long and heavy periods, with vitex for irregular cycles and to enhance fertility, and with cramp bark for dysmenorrhea or painful periods. Red raspberry leaf is of tremendous healing support for many women with fibroids, endometriosis, or heavy, painful, or irregular periods. Along with its uterine-supporting action, red raspberry leaf is also a potent astringent herb useful in the context of hemorrhoids or other prolapse in the pelvic floor.

Active constituents in red raspberry leaf include gallotannins and ellagitannins, flavonoids, fragrine, vitamin C, alcohols, aldehydes, ketones, organic acids, terpenoids, carbohydrates, and glycosides.

Red raspberry leaf is one of those medicinal herbs that are ubiquitous in traditional herbal medicine practice and texts while being mostly unrecognized by science at this time. Scientific studies have looked at the fruit of raspberry and its antioxidant value, but few have been conducted about the leaf. The few studies that looked at the beneficial impact of red rasp-berry leaf on uterine health and pregnancy outcomes delivered neutral results at best.

Traditional herbal knowledge can be defined as a cumulative body of evidence, knowledge, practice, ritual, and belief that evolved via adaptive processes, handed down through the generations by cultural transmission, about the relationship of living beings with one another and their environ-ment. In this way, red raspberry leaf shows up as a trusted herbal ally for uterine health, with or without clinical studies.

The recommended dosage for red raspberry leaf is 4–8 grams of dried leaf in a cup of water infused three times daily. In tincture form, take 1–4 milliliters up to three times daily.

Rose

Rosa spp.

Rose belongs in the Rosaceae family. The part used in intimate herbalism is the flower and petals. Rose is an astringent and heart tonic. Clinical herb-alist Larken Bunce calls rose an euphoriant nervine that is both calming and uplifting.[36] It is also antioxidant.

Roses are a symbol of love and passion. The flowers are an aphrodisiac and open the heart. Rose heals emotional imbalances during events like heartbreak or deep grief. It has uplifting and relaxing effects and promotes emotional balance. Roses with pink and red petals are especially high in bioflavonoids, carotenoids, and anthocyanins.

A 2005 study in Taiwan examined the effect of drinking rose tea on pri-mary dysmenorrhea in adolescent girls. After one, three, and six months, drinking rose tea was associated with lower rates of perceived menstrual pain, anxiety, and distress. The study concluded rose tea is a safe and suit-able treatment for dysmenorrhea in teens.[37]

Roses have been intertwined with humans throughout history, used as symbols in art and religion. The fossil record shows roses have existed for over 35 million years. Rose is used by Pacific Northwest coastal indigenous people for cleansing and protection.

The recommended dosage for rose medicine is 2–4 teaspoons of rose petals per cup of water as an infusion. In tincture form or glycerite, place drops over the tongue as needed. Rose infusion can be added to the bath for healing soaks.

Schisandra

Schisandra chinensis

Schisandra belongs in the Schisandraceae family. The part used for therapeutic purposes is the fruit, a berry. Schisandra berry is an adaptogen, liver-protective, trophorestorative, hormone-balancing, aphrodisiac, general tonic, mild antidepressant, and adrenal tonic herb.

Schisandra berry (*wu wei zi,* which translates as "berry of five flavors") is a staple of Traditional Chinese Medicine. The five flavors refer to its distinct taste: at once sour, salty, bitter, sweet, and pungent. In Traditional Chinese Medicine, a perfectly balanced taste is considered a sign of the harmonizing and naturally balancing qualities that the substance may have on the body as a whole.

Schisandra berry has a strong affinity with the reproductive system and uterus, along with libido, lubrication, and overall sexual desire. One of schisandra's superpowers is its action as a hepatic trophorestorative, acting as a deep liver tonic and builder of hepatic function, supporting detoxification pathways and function in big ways. This is especially relevant as it relates to hormone processing and regulation. Its proven properties run the spectrum from aphrodisiac to adaptogen, and it has strong action on PMS, migraines, and hormonal imbalances.

Schisandra tends to dominate herb formulas and has a history of use as a "single" herb—meaning that when you add schisandra to a blend, it will often take over the taste of the other herbs, and so it is often used on its own. Use it as a tincture, decoction, or syrup and take it every day. I like to blend my schisandra remedies with hibiscus for a pop of bright red color and added astringency.

Active constituents in schisandra berry include schisandrin, triterpenes, polysaccharides, organic acids, quercetin, vitamins C and E, and trace elements. Schisandra contains a variety of lignans, important bioactive compounds responsible for the pharmacological activities of the plant.[38] This therapeutic activity includes its effect on liver protection (prevention of hepatitis, stimulation of liver regeneration, and inhibition of hepatocarcinogenesis).

Schisandra chinensis, also known as the magnolia vine, grows in northern Korea, Japan, China, and adjacent regions of Russia. It has a long history of association with health care as a medicinal plant. Schisandra has been consumed as a longevity tonic and superior herb throughout the history of Chinese civilization. It was first written about in China's first herbal encyclopedia, *Shen Nong Ben Cau Jing,* in the third century BCE.

Schisandra plants share habitat with pandas in the cool mountains of the Upper Yangtze region of China. It grows wild in one of the most biodiverse places on the planet and is wild-harvested by rural villagers—many of them elderly, and many of them women and children—whose medicinal herb foraging may make up as much as 40 percent of household income. When it is done right, wild herb foraging can be sustainable, ethical, and traceable. Schisandra plants also make a nice addition to the medicinal garden as a cultivated plant.

The recommended dosage for schisandra is 150 milliliters of decoction drunk twice a day with meals. In tincture form, take 1–3 milliliters up to three times daily. The powdered fruit or fruit extract (this is what is usually found in pills) can be taken at a dosage of 1–3 grams daily with meals. Schisandra berry can be brewed into wines or teas.

Seaweed

Seaweed and algae include macroalgae, like kelp and dulse, as well as microalgae like spirulina and chlorella. Seaweed is a healing substance as well as a functional food. It is rich in fiber and protein, vitamins, trace minerals, healthy fatty acids, and antioxidants. Popular seaweed like kelp and dulse is traditionally enjoyed as a food in the form of flakes added to soups and stews. Spirulina and chlorella, on the other hand, are most commonly consumed in the form of capsules or tablets. In powder form, they can also be added to smoothies, juices, and other raw food treats.

Seaweed is a simple yet transformative addition to intimate herbalism. Seaweed protects against breast cancer. Many in vivo and in vitro studies of dietary seaweed intake show lower angiogenesis (the splitting and forming of new cancer cells) and increased apoptosis of tumor cells as a result of seaweed consumption. Seaweed inhibits tumor cell adhesion and metastasis while also supporting enhanced immune responses.[39]

Seaweed consumption is also associated with lower rates of heart disease. A healthy heart allows for a healthy sex life and helps prevent erectile dysfunction. Spirulina in particular has been studied for its impact on sexual wellness in the context of obesity. In a 2020 study, spirulina increased the number of erections, reduced latency time between erections, increased nitric oxide bioavailability, and reduced oxidative stress and inflammation.[40]

Chlorella cleanses the body of heavy metals, with potential healing benefits to fertility and healthy reproductive organ function.[41] Finally, seaweed consumption protects against depression and other mood disorders.[42]

Adding healing seaweed and algae to your wellness routine is an easy and nutritious way to enhance sexual and reproductive health. The recommended dosage is 5 grams of dried seaweed per day. For spirulina and chlorella tablets, follow the recommended dosage listed on the bottle.

Shatavari

Asparagus racemosus

Shatavari belongs to the Asparagaceae family. The part used medicinally is the root. Shatavari root is an adaptogenic, uterine tonic, demulcent and emollient, aphrodisiac, antidepressant, and anxiolytic herb.

Shatavari is a staple of Ayurveda and acts as a general tonic. Shatavari is used for reproductive health, hormonal balance, PMS, and the management of menopausal symptoms. For vaginal dryness, shatavari powder is used as a vaginal suppository made with cacao butter and coconut oil to assist with lubrication and to naturally moisten the vaginal membranes.

Shatavari is beneficial in female infertility, increases libido, enhances folliculogenesis and ovulation, prepares the womb for conception, prevents miscarriages, and acts as a postpartum tonic by increasing lactation and toning the uterus postbirth. Shatavari is known as a hormonal herb. The phytoestrogenic activity is due to the presence of steroidal saponins, which exert hormone-like actions in the body, and also due to the isoflavones with mild estrogenic activity that help to balance estrogen levels. Shatavari extract may increase the weight of the ovaries and enhance folliculogenesis.

Active constituents in shatavari include steroidal saponins like shatavarin as well as alkaloids, isoflavones, polysaccharides and mucilage, sterols, trace minerals, and essential fatty acids. Clinical studies on shatavari are still few and far between, especially with human trials. It has been shown to be safe and effective via the herbal tradition over thousands of years of use. A 2011 study on shatavari demonstrated helpful antidepressant effects; for best results, pair shatavari with ashwagandha and holy basil for its antianxiety and antidepressant effects.[43]

Shatavari is common throughout Sri Lanka, India, and the Himalayas.

The recommended dosage for shatavari is 5 grams of powder daily. In tincture form, take 1–3 milliliters up to three times daily. In capsules, take the equivalent of 1,200 milligrams per day.

Tulsi

Ocimum sanctum or *Ocimum tenuiflorum*

Tulsi (also called holy basil; the names are used interchangeably) belongs to the Lamiaceae family. The parts used are the leaf and the aerial parts. Tulsi offers medicinal properties as an adaptogenic, nervine, aphrodisiac, antimicrobial, antioxidant, and immunomodulatory herb.

Tulsi is traditionally used as an adaptogenic herb to promote health and longevity. Tulsi brings many benefits to the body as a whole as a general tonic with a special affinity for stress reduction and liver protection. It makes an excellent herbal tea with a delicious taste and pairs well with other tonics like nettle and milky oats as well as aromatic herbs like mint. For stress reduction, tulsi can be paired with ashwagandha. For liver support, pair tulsi with milk thistle or schisandra.

Tulsi contains alkaloids, carbohydrates, fats, glycosides, phenols, proteins, saponins, tannins, and terpenes. One of its active ingredients is eugenol. A 2008 study showed the beneficial effects of tulsi on stress regulation and relief for anxiety and depression. Thirty-five participants received a 500-milligram tulsi extract capsule twice daily for a period of sixty days. Tulsi proved to be an excellent anxiolytic, and reduced symptoms of generalized anxiety disorder, stress, and depression.[44]

A randomized, double-blind, placebo-controlled study published in 2012 explored the effect of tulsi on stress. The 158 participants showed stress symptoms that included forgetfulness, sexual problems, sleep issues, and feelings of exhaustion and overwork. They received either a placebo or tulsi extract at a dosage of 1,200 milligrams per day for six weeks. The severity of stress-related symptoms was assessed at weeks 0, 2, 4, and 6 of the trial period via a symptom-rating scale. At the six-week mark, there was a significant reduction in stress symptoms in the group who received tulsi compared with placebo. The tulsi group experienced a 39 percent improvement of their general stress symptoms, with no adverse effects.[45]

Tulsi is one of the principal herbs used in the Ayurvedic medicine system, where it is classified as a rasayana (rejuvenating tonic). It holds a supreme place in the ancient Vedic scriptures and is integrated into daily life by Hindus through religious worship. Hindu homes typically have a tulsi plant growing in an earthen pot in or around the home. In Ayurveda, it is believed that the best way to take tulsi medicinally is in its raw, fresh, whole form as a hot-water infusion.

The recommended dosage for tulsi is 1 tablespoon of dried herb per cup of water; drink as needed. In tincture form, take 1–5 milliliters per day. In capsule form, take 500 milligrams up to three times per day.

Vitex

Vitex agnus-castus

Vitex (also called chaste tree, chasteberry, monk's pepper) belongs to the Verbenaceae family. The parts used are the fruit (berries) and leaves. Vitex is a reproductive system tonic, emmenagogue, pituitary adjuvant, carminative, and anti-inflammatory herb.

Traditionally, vitex has been used in the treatment of menstrual disorders, premenstrual syndrome, hyperprolactinemia, infertility, and menopause.[46] Vitex has direct action on both the hypothalamus and the pituitary gland, leading to indirect action on hormone balance. Vitex has a dopaminergic effect on the pituitary gland. The action is vitex binding to dopamine receptors in the pituitary gland, which causes a decrease in prolactin. This then has an effect on other hormones, such as progesterone, which is increased during the luteal phase of the menstrual cycle. Overall, this can decrease the symptoms of PMS, since PMS sufferers tend to have higher levels of prolactin during their cycles. The German Commission E has approved the use of vitex for irregular menstrual cycles, PMS, and mastodynia. Vitex contains phytoestrogens that have an effect on the female reproductive system. Active constituents in vitex include flavonoids, iridoids, volatile oils, linoleic acid, and castine.

A 2014 study conducted with sixty-nine female Japanese participants assessed the efficacy of vitex for the treatment of PMS.[47] Participants took 20 milligrams of vitex extract once per day for the duration of three menstrual cycles. By the end of the first cycle, a significant difference was reported in PMS symptoms. Scores of PMS symptoms continued to decrease significantly over the next two cycles, and the study concluded that vitex is an effective treatment for PMS.

In a double-blind, placebo-controlled pilot study conducted with thirty women of reproductive age, twenty-four to forty-six years old, a supplement containing vitex, green tea, and other nutritional supplements was used in the treatment of infertility.[48] The women had all attempted pregnancy for the six to thirty-six months preceding the trial. After three months, the group using the supplement had an increase in mid-luteal phase progesterone levels and an increase in the number of days during the cycle with increased basal body temperature, indicative of a healthy luteal phase length. After five months of treatment, 33 percent of the supplement group had conceived while none of the placebo group did.

A 2019 study on a group of fifty-two women experiencing menopausal symptoms examined the use of vitex compared to a placebo.[49] After eight weeks, a significant difference was found between the vitex group and the placebo group, which the authors concluded makes vitex a useful herb in the treatment of the symptoms of menopause.

Vitex is a plant native to the Mediterranean region of Europe and Central Asia. It is reported that vitex has been used since Greek and Roman times for treatment of female reproductive disorders. Vitex was referred to both by Hippocrates and Dioscorides for the effect it has on the female reproductive system. The "chaste" in *chasteberry* and *chaste tree* is a name that highlights the plant's reported ability to decrease libido. While there are reports of reduction in libido, this has not been backed up by modern science. What has been backed up is vitex's ability to regulate hormones, particularly with regard to symptoms associated with PMS, including constipation, irritability, depressed mood, migraines, breast tenderness, as well as menopause and infertility.

The recommended dosage for vitex is 175–225 milligrams per day. In tincture form, take 0.2–1 milliliters up to three times per day. Dr. Marisa Marciano warns that high doses of vitex—twenty times the recommended therapeutic dosage—can inhibit all aspects of anterior pituitary function, resulting in decreased pituitary, adrenal, and uterine function.

8

Intimate Herbal Recipes

NETTLE AND MILKY OATS INFUSION

Nettle and milky oats infusion is the starting point for many protocols in the intimate herbal practice. This infusion is a safe, yummy, and deeply restorative tonic for anyone looking to support their sexual and reproductive health with the help of herbs.

Nettle is a functional herb that acts as a general tonic, while milky oats deeply replenish a tired nervous system. It provides essential vitamins and minerals along with active compounds that act as adaptogenic and rejuvenating herbs to enhance body function as a whole, with special affinity for nervous system support, stable energy levels, a healthy libido, and sexual vitality.

This infusion is safe to drink, even in large amounts. Drink up to 4 cups daily. As a slow and steady builder, this is an herbal remedy well suited to daily long-term use. To jazz up the recipe, you can add peppermint, hibiscus, fennel seeds, ginger, or other delicious aromatic herbs.

> 1 cup water
> 1 Tbsp. dried nettle leaf
> 1 Tbsp. dried milky oats

Bring the water to a boil, remove from heat, and add the dried nettle leaf and the dried milky oats.

Let steep for 10–20 minutes, strain, and enjoy.

ELEUTHERO AND SCHISANDRA DECOCTION

For roots and berries, decoctions are better than infusions at extracting healing compounds. The eleuthero and schisandra decoction offers deep nourishment and adaptogen support.

Eleuthero gives energy support while schisandra strongly nourishes the liver. As a tonifying remedy intended for ongoing, regular, and steady use, it can be used as a base for elixir-making when blended with yummy delectable oils or fats like coconut oil or cacao butter. Blend it with honey or another sweetener, chai tea, ginger infusion, or even bone broth. The possibilities are wide and varied.

When I make a big batch of this decoction, I like to freeze it into ice cube trays for later use. You can pop them in the blender with smoothies or fresh juices for a quick and easy adaptogenic herbal brew. Drink 1 cup daily.

1 cup water
1 Tbsp. schisandra berry
1 Tbsp. eleuthero root

Combine 1 Tbsp. of schisandra berry and 1 Tbsp. of eleuthero root in a stockpot for every cup of water you intend to use. For decoctions, I recommend using at least 1 quart of liquid per recipe, because some of the water will evaporate during simmering. I usually make decoctions in 4-quart batches.

Cover your pot and bring to a boil over the stove.

Reduce heat and allow to simmer for 30–60 minutes.

Remove from the heat and leave to cool, covered, before straining.

CACAO, MACA, AND ASHWAGANDHA ELIXIR

This yummy blend tastes as good as hot chocolate but delivers the fertility-boosting, hormone-balancing, and mind-calming effects of adaptogenic herbs along with increased focus and stamina from cacao. Maca has a sweet malty flavor that pairs well with cacao.

Ashwagandha is commonly enjoyed in warm milk in Ayurvedic tradition, and I adore its earthy taste combined with milk and honey. This blend makes a great morning herbal sip to encourage energy and focus. As a nourishing drink, it can be enjoyed daily. For a nighttime elixir, remove the cacao and maca and enjoy ashwagandha blended in the warm tonic drink.

MAKES 2 SERVINGS

1½ cups warm milk or plant-based milk
2 Tbsp. cacao powder
1 Tbsp. maca
1 Tbsp. ashwagandha powder
1 Tbsp. coconut oil
1 tsp. honey
¼ tsp. vanilla extract
pinch high-quality sea salt

Combine all the ingredients in a high-speed blender. Blend for 20–30 seconds or until creamy and frothy.

If desired, you can add a dropperful of ashwagandha tincture or maca tincture to your serving glass.

SCHISANDRA AND ROSE ELIXIR

Delicious served hot or cold over ice, the schisandra and rose elixir offers a bright pink cup of heart medicine boosted by the aphrodisiac properties of schisandra berry. For an even brighter pop of color, add a teaspoon of dried beet powder or a splash of hibiscus tea. Schisandra is a fantastic daily herbal support for healthy hormones and a well-functioning liver. Schisandra and rose together make the skin glow and nourish the heart. This elixir can be enjoyed daily.

MAKES 2 SERVINGS

1½ cups water, hot or cold
1 Tbsp. rose hydrosol
1 Tbsp. coconut oil
1 tsp. honey (if you have rose-infused honey on hand, use it)

½ tsp. schisandra extract powder
¼ tsp. vanilla extract
pinch high-quality sea salt

Combine all the ingredients in a high-speed blender. Blend for 20–30 seconds or until creamy and frothy.

If desired, add a dropperful of schisandra tincture or rose elixir to your serving glass. Enjoy!

WILD ROSE ELIXIR

Roses are incredibly beautiful flowers that carry with them a symbol of love, romance, and sensuality. With over 150 different species along with thousands of hybrids, roses are among nature's most exquisite creations, with their full, delicate blooms, intoxicating fragrance, and lush foliage.

This elixir is best made with fresh wild roses when they are in bloom. Be sure to pick them in a wholesome environment from rose bushes that haven't been sprayed with pesticides or herbicides, which is common in city areas and on city land. Harvest the rose petals or rosebuds into a small basket or cloth cotton bag, making sure to leave plenty of blooms on the bush for the pollinators as well as to ensure renewed growth for generations to come.

1 part honey
1 part brandy
1 part fresh wild rose

At home, clean the petals and remove any pieces of leaves, insects, or other plant parts.

Fill a clean glass jar with the rose petals and cover with half brandy, half honey.

Other liquid sweeteners also blend well with a rose elixir, including molasses, maple syrup, and vegetable glycerin.

Close the lid, give it a good shake, and place in the pantry for 2–4 weeks.

Strain and bottle your elixir into small amber-colored bottles with droppers, and enjoy.

GINGER AND ROSEMARY SYRUP

A circulation enhancer, this syrup warms the body, supports digestion, and enhances blood flow. Use this syrup as an addition to any sparkling water, kombucha, cocktail, or drink for its action as a circulatory tonic and delicious taste. You can also use this recipe as a base for other syrups, or start with a decoction of berries and roots to reduce down into a syrupy herb brew. Enjoy up to 2 tablespoons per day.

4 Tbsp. fresh ginger, or 2 Tbsp. powdered
4 Tbsp. fresh rosemary, or 2 Tbsp. dried
4 cups water
1 cup honey
dropperfuls of tincture: ginger, rosemary, *Ginkgo biloba*,
or ginseng

Combine the ginger, rosemary, and water in a pot.

Cover and bring to a boil.

Reduce heat to low and let simmer for 10–20 minutes.

Remove from heat and strain into a smaller pot.

Place back on the stove at medium heat, uncovered, and reduce the liquid down to half its original volume.

When it's down to about a cup of liquid, add honey and stir to dissolve.

Let cool completely before bottling. Then pour syrup into bottles and label. Store in the refrigerator for up to six months.

Optional: Add 1 part tincture to 3 parts syrup for an herbal boost and longer shelf life.

HIBISCUS AND DAMIANA SYRUP

A mood-lifting blend, hibiscus delivers a refreshing pop of color that brightens any day, while damiana acts as a potent aphrodisiac and antidepressant for low moods and anxiety. A delicious-tasting recipe, this syrup will easily accommodate less palatable medicinals, so feel free to add extracts from ashwagandha or reishi for extra potency. Enjoy up to 2 tablespoons per day.

4 Tbsp. hibiscus
2 Tbsp. damiana
4 cups water
1 cup honey
dropperfuls of tincture: ashwagandha, reishi, schisandra, or damiana

Combine the hibiscus, damiana, and water in a pot.

Cover and bring to a boil.

Reduce heat to low and let simmer for 10–20 minutes.

Remove from heat and strain into a smaller pot.

Place back on the stove at medium heat, uncovered, and reduce the liquid down to half its original volume.

When it's down to about a cup of liquid, add honey and stir to dissolve.

Let cool completely before bottling. Then pour syrup into bottles and label. Store in the refrigerator for up to six months.

Optional: Add 1 part tincture to 3 parts syrup for an herbal boost and longer shelf life.

CACAO, CARDAMOM, ORANGE, AND DAMIANA WINE

I like to make this herbal recipe with white wine, but red wine, rosé, and orange wine could be substituted as well. The cacao nibs, cracked cardamom pods, dried orange peel, and dried damiana leaf all come together to make a heartwarming, stimulating beverage that enhances digestion and boosts libido.

1 bottle (750 milliliters) white wine
2 Tbsp. cacao nibs

1 Tbsp. cracked cardamom pods
1 Tbsp. dried orange peel
1 Tbsp. dried damiana leaf

Combine all ingredients together in the wine bottle.

Place in the fridge for 10–14 days to infuse.

Strain and enjoy up to 1 glass per day.

OAT STRAW AND DAMIANA HERBAL BATH

Deeply soothing and restorative to the nervous system, this bath blend with oat straw and damiana smells heavenly and is the perfect gateway to a gentle, sensual moment. Oat straw acts as a deeply restorative nervous system tonic, while damiana is a nervine, antidepressant, and aphrodisiac with delightful woody and floral aromas.

2 cups dried oat straw
2 cups dried damiana
4 quarts water

Prepare a warm bath.

In a large stockpot over the stove, place 4 quarts of water and add the oat straw and damiana.

Cover and bring to a boil.

Reduce heat and let simmer for 15–30 minutes.

Strain into a large bowl and pour into the bath. Enjoy!

Tip: The same herbs can be reinfused up to four times in your stockpot.

HEALING BREAST OIL

Blending together potent lymphatics and anti-inflammatory herbs, breast oil applied as a gentle massage keeps the breasts supple and healthy. Plantain leaf is a healing emollient to keep the skin nourished, while cleavers and calendula act as deeply potent lymphatic tonic herbs.

1 clean glass jar with a tight-fitting lid
plantain leaf, gently wilted or dried
cleavers aerial parts, gently wilted or dried
calendula flower, gently wilted or dried
oil to cover: olive, sunflower, or fractionated coconut oil
optional: essential oils such as rose or rosemary

Place the wilted herbs in the glass jar and add oil to cover, ensuring the herbs are fully submerged.

Close the lid and place the jar in the pantry or other dark place to infuse for 2 weeks.

Strain and bottle. Apply on the breast for breast massage.

HEALING BREAST SALVE

To turn the healing breast oil into a salve:

healing breast oil
beeswax

Measure the herbal oil and use a ¼ ratio of beeswax to oil: If you have 1 cup oil, use ¼ cup beeswax.

Combine oil and beeswax in a pot and gently warm to dissolve.

Stir, pour into small salve jars.

Let cool completely before closing the lid.

SCHISANDRA TINCTURE

Use this recipe as a template for liquid extracts and tinctures in alcohol, vinegar, or glycerin. Swap schisandra berries for other herbs like dandelion root, hawthorn berries, and others. Here, schisandra is extracted into alcohol to make a daily tincture for liver support, migraine relief, healthy hormones, and a strong libido.

1 clean glass jar with a tight-fitting lid
whole dried schisandra berries
alcohol to cover, such as brandy or vodka

Fill the jar to ⅓ with schisandra berries.

Add alcohol to cover, ensuring the berries are fully submerged.

Close the lid and place your jar in the pantry or other dark place to infuse for 4 weeks.

Strain and bottle.

ADAPTOGENIC CHOCOLATE BARK

Eating medicinal herbs in cacao is the best vessel for healing, sensual remedies. You can switch up your herbs every time you make a batch of this delicious chocolate bark. Adaptogenic herbs lend themselves well to this recipe, as they can be enjoyed daily for a deep tonic effect. Maca and ashwagandha pair deliciously well with cacao. Additional toppings include pollen, schisandra berry powder, and edible flowers.

FOR THE BARK:
1 cup cacao butter
1 cup cacao powder
½ cup coconut sugar or honey
optional: pinch high-quality sea salt

Combine all ingredients in a double boiler and gently melt to dissolve.

For a medicinal chocolate bark base, add 1–2 tsp. herb powder (ashwagandha, maca, shatavari).

Pour the blend on a baking sheet covered with parchment paper and let cool. The bark will harden as it cools.

FOR TOPPINGS:

ginger, cayenne, ashwagandha, maca, shatavari, schisandra berry, reishi, or eleuthero powders

flower petals from calendula, rose, violet, borage, or other edible flowers

pine pollen, lotus pollen, or bee pollen

Sprinkle the powders over the bark as it cools.

Flower petals can be added.

Dust with pollen.

Notes

Introduction

1 Caffyn Jesse, "Elements of Intimacy: The Dance of Loving Connection," *EroSpirit*. Independently published. July 4, 2019.

1. Foundations of Intimate Herbalism

1 Sophie Duncan, "Critical Relationality: Queer, Indigenous, and Multispecies Belonging Beyond Settler Sex & Nature," *Imaginations,* July 25, 2019. doi:10.17742/IMAGE.CR.10.1.4. https://tinyurl.com/4r5y8x4s.

2 Amanda Karst, "Conservation Value of the North American Boreal Forest from an Ethnobotanical Perspective," Canadian Boreal Initiative, 2010. https://tinyurl.com/7ed746vu.

3 Biljana Bauer Petrovska, "Historical Review of Medicinal Plants' Usage," *Pharmacognosy Reviews* 6:11 (January 2012), 1–5. doi:10.4103/0973-7847.95849.

4 N. H. Aboelsoud, "Herbal Medicine in Ancient Egypt," *Journal of Medicinal Plants Research* 4:2 (December 8, 2009), 82–86. doi:10.5897/JMPR09.013.

5 Rajesh Nair, Senthy Sellaturay, and Seshadri Sriprasad, "The History of Ginseng in the Management of Erectile Dysfunction in Ancient China (3500–2600 BCE)," *Indian Journal of Urology* 28:1 (January 2012), 15–20. doi:10.4103/0970-1591.94946.

6 Nagendra Singh Chauhan et al., "A Review on Plants Used for Improvement of Sexual Performance and Virility," *Biomed Research International* 2014 (August 18, 2014). doi:10.1155/2014/868062.

7 John M. Riddle and J. Worth Estes, "Oral Contraceptives in Ancient and Medieval Times," *American Scientist* 80:3 (May 1992). doi:10.2307/29774642.

8 Ember Peters, "Wild Carrot Monograph," *Wild Current Herbalism,* December 2014.

9 Victoria Sweet, "Hildegard of Bingen and the Greening of Medieval Medicine," *Bulletin of the History of Medicine* 73:3 (Fall 1999), 381–403. doi:10.1353/bhm.1999.0140.

10 Jeff Wallenfeldt, "Salem Witch Trials: History & Causes," *Encyclopedia Britannica,* n.d. www.britannica.com/event/Salem-witch-trials.

11 Bob Cole, "'The Very Future of Our Nations': How Aboriginal Midwifery Represents a Practical Model for Utilization of Traditional Knowledge," *Journal of Integrated Studies* 10:1 (2018). https://tinyurl.com/th9x776r.

12 E. Richard Brown, *Rockefeller Medicine Men: Medicine and Capitalism in America* (Berkeley, CA: University of California Press, 1979).

13 James C. Whorton, "Cultism to CAM: The Flexner Report Reconsidered," *Complementary Health Practice Review* 6:2 (Winter–Spring 2001).

14 Rosita Arvigo, "My Mentors," November 9, 2020. https://rositaarvigo.com /about/my-mentors.

15 Michael J. Balick and Hugh O'Brien, "Ethnobotanical and Floristic Research in Belize: Accomplishments, Challenges and Lessons Learned," *Ethnobotany Research and Applications* 2 (2004), 77–88. https://tinyurl.com/3knmrze9.

16 Arvigo, "My Mentors."

2. When Not to Use Herbs

1 Larken Bunce, "Herbs and Somatic Practices for Stress, Trauma and Resilience," Dandelion Seed Conference, Olympia, WA, 2017. https://tinyurl.com /42ephxtj.

2 Annie Sprinkle and Beth Stephens, "Ecosexuality: The Story of Our Love with the Earth," in *Assuming the Ecosexual Position: The Earth as Lover* (Chicago: University of Chicago Press, 2021).

3 Irwin Goldstein, "The Central Mechanisms of Sexual Function," Boston University School of Medicine, February 7, 2003. https://tinyurl.com/w4any5bd.

4 Becky K. Lynn et al., "The Relationship between Marijuana Use Prior to Sex and Sexual Function in Women," *Sexual Medicine* 7:2 (June 1, 2019), 192–97. doi:10.1016/j.esxm.2019.01.003.

5 Francesc Borrell-Carrió, Anthony L. Suchman, and Ronald M. Epstein, "The Biopsychosocial Model 25 Years Later: Principles, Practice, and Scientific Inquiry," *Annals of Family Medicine* 2:6 (2004), 576–82. doi:10.1370/afm.245.

6 Vicki Brower, "Mind-body Research Moves Towards the Mainstream," *European Molecular Biology Organization Reports* 7:4 (2006), 358–61. doi:10.1038 /sj.embor.7400671.

7 American Psychological Association, "Stress Effects on the Body," November 1, 2018. www.apa.org/topics/stress/body.

8 Elizabeth Williamson, Samuel Driver, and Karen Baxter, eds., *Stockley's Herbal Medicines Interactions* (Chicago: Pharmaceutical Press, 2009). https://tinyurl.com/2tcnukwp.

9 National Center for Complementary and Integrative Health, "Herb-Drug Interactions," *NCCIH Clinical Digest,* September 2015. https://tinyurl.com/skamjkb2.

10 Williamson et al., *Stockley's Herbal Medicines Interactions.*

3. Becoming an Intimate Herbalist

1 European Medicines Agency, "Assessment Report on *Avena sativa* L., Herba and *Avena sativa* L., Fructus," September 4, 2008. https://tinyurl.com/6j645hr7.

2 Rachel H. X. Wong et al., "Chronic Effects of a Wild Green Oat Extract Supplementation on Cognitive Performance in Older Adults: A Randomised, Double-Blind, Placebo-Controlled, Crossover Trial," *Nutrients* 4:5 (May 1, 2012), 331–42. doi:10.3390/nu4050331.

3 Michael Wink, "Modes of Action of Herbal Medicines and Plant Secondary Metabolites," *Medicines (Basel)* 2:3 (September 1, 2015), 251–86. doi:10.3390/medicines2030251.

4 Anne Stobart, "The Working of Herbs, Part 5: Medicinal Herb Constituents and Actions," The Recipes Project, January 7, 2014. https://recipes.hypotheses.org/3076.

5 Abdullahi R. Abubakar and Mainul Haque, "Preparation of Medicinal Plants: Basic Extraction and Fractionation Procedures for Experimental Purposes," *Journal of Pharmacy and Bioallied Sciences* 12:1 (January–March 2020), 1–10. doi:10.4103/jpbs.JPBS_175_19.

6 Glen Nagel, "Mastering Menstruums in Herbal Extracts," Traditional Roots Conference, Portland, OR, 2017. https://tinyurl.com/2f9kbs3h.

4. The Intimate Herbal Pharmacy

1 V. Beck, U. Rohr, and A. Jungbauer, "Phytoestrogens Derived from Red Clover: An Alternative to Estrogen Replacement Therapy?" *Journal of Steroid Biochemistry and Molecular Biology* 94:5 (March 23, 2005), 499–518. doi:10.1016/j.jsbmb.2004.12.038.

2 Patrick E. McGovern, Armen Mirzoian, and Gretchen R. Hall, "Ancient Egyptian Herbal Wines," *Proceedings of the National Academy of Sciences* 106:18 (May 5, 2009), 7361–66. doi:10.1073/pnas.0811578106.

5. Sexual and Reproductive Health

1   Adam Safron, "What Is Orgasm? A Model of Sexual Trance and Climax Via Rhythmic Entrainment," *Socioaffective Neuroscience and Psychology* 6 (October 25, 2016). doi:10.3402/snp.v6.31763.

2   Kara Sigler, "TransNatural for Professionals," American Herbalists Guild, n.d. https://tinyurl.com/226ty87u.

6. Intimate Health Conditions

1   Roger Pamphlett et al., "Elemental Bioimaging Shows Mercury and Other Toxic Metals in Normal Breast Tissue and in Breast Cancers," *PloS One,* January 31, 2020. doi:10.1371/journal.pone.0228226.

2   Whitecoat Strategies, "Premenstrual Breast Pain Is Reduced with Red Clover Supplement," Whitecoat Strategies, Washington, DC, November 15, 2001. https://tinyurl.com/xpecejv7.

3   Charlotte Atkinson et al., "Red Clover–Derived Isoflavones and Mammographic Breast Density: A Double-Blind, Randomized, Placebo-Controlled Trial," *Breast Cancer Research* 6:R170–79 (February 24, 2004). doi:10.1186/bcr773.

4   Trevor J. Powles et al., "Red Clover Isoflavones Are Safe and Well Tolerated in Women with a Family History of Breast Cancer," *Journal of the British Menopause Society* 14:1 (March 2008), 6–12. doi:10.1258/mi.2007.007033.

5   Hua Luo et al., "Naturally Occurring Anticancer Compounds: Shining from Chinese Herbal Medicine," *Chinese Medicine* 14:48 (2019). doi:10.1186/s13020-019-0270-9.

6   Ibid.

7   Ibid.

8   Ibid.

9   Science Direct, "Astragalus," 2018. https://tinyurl.com/3tuddpt2.

10 Meriem Koual et al., "Environmental Chemicals, Breast Cancer Progression and Drug Resistance," *Environmental Health* 19:117 (2020). doi:10.1186/s12940-020-00670-2.

11 Brandi Patrice Smith and Zeynep Madak-Erdogan, "Urban Neighborhood and Residential Factors Associated with Breast Cancer in African American Women: A Systematic Review," *Hormones and Cancer* 9 (2018), 71–81. doi:10.1007/s12672-018-0325-x.

12 Guo-Shiou Liao, Maria Karmella Apaya, and Lie-Fen Shyur, "Herbal Medicine and Acupuncture for Breast Cancer Palliative Care and Adjuvant Therapy," *Complementary and Alternative Medicine* 2013:437948. doi:10.1155/2013/437948.

13 Biswa Mohan Biswal et al., "Effect of *Withania somnifera* (Ashwagandha) on the Development of Chemotherapy-Induced Fatigue and Quality of Life in Breast Cancer Patients," *Integrative Cancer Therapies* 12:4 (July 2013), 312–22. doi:10.1177/1534735412464551.

14 Mariann Garner-Wizard et al., "Adjunct Treatment with Ashwagandha Root Extract for Fatigue from Chemotherapy for Breast Cancer," *HerbClip* June 14, 2013. https://tinyurl.com/6cv2zuf4.

15 Liao et al., "Herbal Medicine and Acupuncture."

16 Ibid.

17 Hong Zhao et al., "Spore Powder of *Ganoderma lucidum* Improves Cancer-Related Fatigue in Breast Cancer Patients Undergoing Endocrine Therapy: A Pilot Clinical Trial," *Complementary and Alternative Medicine* 2012:809614. doi:10.1155/2012/809614.

18 Liao et al., "Herbal Medicine and Acupuncture."

19 Hiva Alipanah, Mohammad Reza Bigdeli, and Mohammad Ali Esmaeili, "Inhibitory Effect of *Viola odorata* Extract on Tumor Growth and Metastasis in 4T1 Breast Cancer Model," *Iranian Journal of Pharmaceutical Research* 17:1 (Winter 2018), 276–91. https://tinyurl.com/3u4pbskn.

20 Harika Atmaca et al., "Effects of *Galium aparine* Extract on the Cell Viability, Cell Cycle and Cell Death in Breast Cancer Cell Lines," *Journal of Ethnopharmacology* 186 (June 20, 2016), 305–10. doi:10.1016/j.jep.2016.04.007.

21 Charlotte Wessel Skovlund et al., "Association of Hormonal Contraception with Depression," *JAMA Psychiatry* 73:11 (November 2016), 1154–62. doi:10.1001/jamapsychiatry.2016.2387.

22 Patricia A. Murphy et al., "Interaction of St. John's Wort with Oral Contraceptives: Effects on the Pharmacokinetics of Norethindrone and Ethinyl Estradiol, Ovarian Activity and Breakthrough Bleeding," *Contraception* 71:6 (June 2005), 402–8. doi:10.1016/j.contraception.2004.11.004.

23 Evidence-Based Medicine Consult, "Medication & Herbal Inhibitors of the Cytochrome P450 (CYP) Enzymes Drug Table," n.d. https://tinyurl.com/5xnvsjdb.

24 Nick H. Mashour, George I. Lin, and William H. Frishman, "Herbal Medicine for the Treatment of Cardiovascular Disease," *Archives of Internal Medicine* 158:20 (1998), 2225–34. doi:10.1001/archinte.158.20.2225.

25 National Institute of Diabetes and Digestive and Kidney Diseases, "Estrogens and Oral Contraceptives," in *LiverTox: Clinical and Research Information on Drug-Induced Liver Injury,* May 28, 2020. https://tinyurl.com/36xw6cvd.

26 Robin Rose Bennett, "Wild Carrot Exploration," Herbal Medicine and EarthSpirit Teachings, August 2011. https://tinyurl.com/4taafvf9.

27 *Integrative Herbalism,* Summer 2014 issue, Vermont Center for Integrative Herbalism. https://tinyurl.com/4wskv73p.

28 Johnna Nynas et al., "Depression and Anxiety Following Early Pregnancy Loss: Recommendations for Primary Care Providers," *Primary Care Companion to CNS Disorders* 17:1 (2015). doi:10.4088/PCC.14r01721.

29 *Integrative Herbalism,* Summer 2014.

30 Sai Kong et al., "The Complementary and Alternative Medicine for Endometriosis: A Review of Utilization and Mechanism," *Complementary and Alternative Medicine* 2014:146383. doi:10.1155/2014/146383.

31 Antonio Simone Laganà et al., "Anxiety and Depression in Patients with Endometriosis: Impact and Management Challenges," *International Journal of Women's Health* 9 (2017), 323–30. doi:10.2147/IJWH.S119729.

32 Sherry Rier and Warren G. Foster, "Environmental Dioxins and Endometriosis," *Toxicological Sciences* 70:2 (December 2002), 161–70. doi:10.1093/toxsci/70.2.161.

33 Kong et al., "Complementary and Alternative Medicine"; Laganà et al., "Anxiety and Depression."

34 Kong et al., "Complementary and Alternative Medicine."

35 Mert Ilhan, Fatma Tuğçe Gürağaç Dereli, and Esra Küpeli Akkol, "Novel Drug Targets with Traditional Herbal Medicines for Overcoming Endometriosis," *Current Drug Delivery* 16:5 (June 2019), 386–99. doi:10.2174/1567201816666181227112421.

36 Alexandre Vallée and Yves Lecarpentier, "Curcumin and Endometriosis," *International Journal of Molecular Sciences* 21:7 (April 2020), 2440. doi:10.3390/ijms21072440.

37 Weilin Zheng et al., "Anti-Angiogenic Alternative and Complementary Medicines for the Treatment of Endometriosis: A Review of Potential Molecular Mechanisms," *Complementary and Alternative Medicine* 2018:4128984. doi:10.1155/2018/4128984.

38 Kong et al., "Complementary and Alternative Medicine."

39 Sheyda Jouhari et al., "Effects of Silymarin, Cabergoline and Letrozole on Rat Model of Endometriosis," *Taiwanese Journal of Obstetrics and Gynecology* 57:6 (December 2018), 830–35. doi:10.1016/j.tjog.2018.10.011.

40 Cristina Lull, Harry J. Wichers, and Huub F. J. Savelkoul, "Anti-inflammatory and Immunomodulating Properties of Fungal Metabolites," *Mediators of Inflammation* 2005:2 (June 9, 2005), 63–80. doi:10.1155/MI.2005.63.

41 Paolo Capogrosso et al., "One Patient Out of Four with Newly Diagnosed Erectile Dysfunction Is a Young Man—Worrisome Picture from the Everyday Clinical Practice," *Journal of Sexual Medicine* 10:7 (2013). doi:10.1111/jsm.12179.

42 U.S. Centers for Disease Control and Prevention, "*Health, United States* Spotlight: Racial and Ethnic Disparities in Heart Disease," April 2019. https://tinyurl.com/4p2zx68t.

43 Roland Dyck et al., "Epidemiology of Diabetes Mellitus among First Nations and Non–First Nations Adults," *Canadian Medical Association Journal* 182:3 (February 2010), 249–56. doi:10.1503/cmaj.090846.

44 Sean A. Martin et al., "Predictors of Sexual Dysfunction Incidence and Remission in Men," *Journal of Sexual Medicine* 11:5 (May 1, 2014), 1136–47. doi:10.1111/jsm.12483.

45 Hye Won Lee et al., "Ginseng for Erectile Dysfunction," *Cochrane Database of Systematic Reviews* 2017:5 (May 2017), CD012654. doi:10.1002/14651858.CD012654.

46 Byung-Cheul Shin et al., "Maca *(L. meyenii)* for Improving Sexual Function: A Systematic Review," *BMC Complementary and Alternative Medicine* 2010:10, 44. doi:10.1186/1472-6882-10-44.

47 Christina M. Dording, "Safety and Effectiveness Study of Maca Root to Treat Antidepressant-Induced Sexual Dysfunction," ClinicalTrials.gov, 2019. https://tinyurl.com/utayy3yr.

48 An Xiao et al., "Drug-Induced Liver Injury Due to *Lepidium meyenii* (Maca) Medicinal Liquor," *Chinese Medical Journal* 130:24 (December 20, 2017), 3005–6. doi:10.4103/0366-6999.220314.

49 Anna Kessler et al., "The Global Prevalence of Erectile Dysfunction: A Review," *BJU International* 124:4 (October 2019), 587–99. doi:10.1111/bju.14813.

50 A. J. Cohen and B. Bartlik, "*Ginkgo biloba* for Antidepressant-Induced Sexual Dysfunction," *Journal of Sex and Marital Therapy* 24:2 (April–June 1998), 139–43. doi:10.1080/00926239808404927.

51 Forouzan Mohammadi et al., "Effects of Herbal Medicine on Male Infertility," *Anatomical Sciences Journal* 10:4 (November 2013). https://tinyurl.com/y26mycue.

52 Claudia Pivonello et al., "Bisphenol A: An Emerging Threat to Female Fertility," *Reproductive Biology and Endocrinology* 18:22 (2020). doi:10.1186/s12958-019-0558-8.

53 Hareram Birla et al., "Neuroprotective Effects of *Withania somnifera* in BPA-Induced Cognitive Dysfunction and Oxidative Stress in Mice," *Behavioral and Brain Functions* 15:1 (May 7, 2019). https://tinyurl.com/8h2zmk5c; Satyakumar Vidyashankar et al., "Ashwagandha *(Withania somnifera)* Supercritical CO_2 Extract Derived Withanolides Mitigates Bisphenol A Induced Mitochondrial Toxicity in HepG2 Cells," *Toxicology Reports* (Ireland) 1 (July 4, 2014), 1004–12. doi:10.1016/j.toxrep.2014.06.008.

54 E. F. Galimova, Z. K. Amirova, and S. N. Galimov, "Dioxins in the Semen of Men with Infertility," *Environmental Science and Pollution Research International* 22:19 (October 2015), 14566–69. doi:10.1007/s11356-014-3109-z.

55 Peter Simsa et al., "Increased Exposure to Dioxin-like Compounds Is Associated with Endometriosis in a Case-Control Study in Women," *Reproductive Biomedicine Online* 20 (2010), 681–88. doi:10.1016/j.rbmo.2010.01.018. https://tinyurl.com/rj7n9u3n.

56 In Young Bae, Bo-Yeon Kwak, and Hyeon Gyu Lee, "Synergistic Antiradical Action of Natural Antioxidants and Herbal Mixture for Preventing Dioxin Toxicity," *Food Science and Biotechnology* 21 (2012), 491–96. doi:10.1007/s10068-012-0062-9.

57 Park Ki-moon, Hwang Jin-guk, and Kim Hyun-seok, "An Oriental Herb Extracts Composition Having Detoxification Effect on the Nicotine and Dioxin," patent by Hyunseok Kim, filed September 5, 2003, application granted November 8, 2005. https://patents.google.com/patent/KR100526760B1/en.

58 N. Defarge, J. Spiroux de Vendômois, and G. E. Séralini, "Toxicity of Formulants and Heavy Metals in Glyphosate-Based Herbicides and Other Pesticides," *Toxicology Reports* 5 (2018), 156–63. doi:10.1016/j.toxrep.2017.12.025.

59 Reza Mehrandish, Aliasghar Rahimian, and Alireza Shahriary, "Heavy Metals Detoxification: A Review of Herbal Compounds for Chelation Therapy in Heavy Metals Toxicity," *Journal of Herbmed Pharmacology* 8:2 (2019), 69–77. doi:10.15171/jhp.2019.12.

60 Mohaddese Mahboubi and Mona Mahboubi, "Hepatoprotection by Dandelion *(Taraxacum officinale)* and Mechanisms," *Asian Pacific Journal of Tropical Biomedicine* 10:1 (2020), 1–10. doi:10.4103/2221-1691.273081.

61 Williamson et al., *Stockley's Herbal Medicines Interactions*.

62 Huijuan Cao et al., "Can Chinese Herbal Medicine Improve Outcomes of In Vitro Fertilization? A Systematic Review and Meta-Analysis of Randomized Controlled Trials," *PLoS One* 8:12 (2013), e81650. doi:10.1371/journal.pone.0081650.

63 Nava Ainehchi et al., "The Effectiveness of Herbal Mixture Supplements with and without Clomiphene Citrate in Comparison to Clomiphene Citrate on Serum Antioxidants and Glycemic Biomarkers in Women with Polycystic Ovary Syndrome Willing to Be Pregnant: A Randomized Clinical Trial," *Biomolecules* 9:6 (June 2019), 215. doi:10.3390/biom9060215.

64 Rachel Cusatis et al., "Too Much Time? Time Use and Fertility-specific Quality of Life among Men and Women Seeking Specialty Care for Infertility," *BMC Psychology* 7:45 (2019). doi:10.1186/s40359-019-0312-1; Meng-Hsing Wu et al., "Quality of Life among Infertile Women with Endometriosis Undergoing IVF Treatment and Their Pregnancy Outcomes," *Journal of Psychosomatic Obstetrics & Gynecology* 42:1 (2021). doi:10.1080/0167482X.2020.1758659; Meng-Hsing Wu et al., "Quality of Life and Pregnancy Outcomes among Women Undergoing In Vitro Fertilization Treatment: A Longitudinal Cohort Study," *Journal of the Formosan Medical Association* 119:1 (January 2020), 471–79. doi:10.1016/j.jfma.2019.06.015.

65 Kathy Abascal and Eric Yarnell, "Botanical Treatments for Hemorrhoids," *Alternative and Complementary Therapies* 11:6 (December 2005), 285–89. doi:10.1089/act.2005.11.285.

66 Lisa Dawn Hamilton, Alessandra H. Rellini, and Cindy M. Meston, "Cortisol, Sexual Arousal, and Affect in Response to Sexual Stimuli," *Journal of Sexual Medicine* 5:9 (September 2008), 2111–18. doi:10.1111/j.1743-6109.2008.00922.x.

67 K. Chandrasekhar, Jyoti Kapoor, and Sridhar Anishetty, "A Prospective, Randomized Double-Blind, Placebo-Controlled Study of Safety and Efficacy of a High-Concentration Full-Spectrum Extract of Ashwagandha Root in Reducing Stress and Anxiety in Adults," *Indian Journal of Psychological Medicine* 34:3 (July–September 2012), 255–62. doi:10.4103/0253-7176.106022.

68 Khaled G. Abdel-Wahhab et al., "Role of Ashwagandha Methanolic Extract in the Regulation of Thyroid Profile in Hypothyroidism Modeled Rats," *Molecular Biology Reports* 46 (2019), 3637–49. doi:10.1007/s11033-019-04721-x.

69 Adrian L. Lopresti, Peter D. Drummond, and Stephen J. Smith, "A Randomized, Double-Blind, Placebo-Controlled, Crossover Study Examining the Hormonal and Vitality Effects of Ashwagandha *(Withania somnifera)* in Aging, Overweight Males," *American Journal of Men's Health* 13:2 (March–April 2019). doi:10.1177/1557988319835985.

70 Nerea M. Casado-Espada et al., "Hormonal Contraceptives, Female Sexual Dysfunction, and Managing Strategies: A Review," *Journal of Clinical Medicine* 8:6 (June 2019), 908. doi:10.3390/jcm8060908.

71 G. S. Shankar, "Serotonin and Sexual Dysfunction," *Journal of Autacoids and Hormones* 5 (2015), e129. doi:10.4172/2161-0479.1000e129.

72 F. Giuliano and J. Allard, "Dopamine and Sexual Function," *International Journal of Impotence Research* Suppl. 3 (August 13, 2001), S18–28. doi:10.1038/sj.ijir.3900719.

73 Agnes Higgins, Michael Nash, and Aileen M. Lynch, "Antidepressant-Associated Sexual Dysfunction: Impact, Effects, and Treatment," *Drug, Healthcare and Patient Safety* 2 (2010), 141–50. doi:10.2147/DHPS.S7634.

74 Microbicide Trials Network, "Cell Damage Caused by Use of Certain Personal Lubricants Does Not Increase HIV Risk, Lab Study Finds," *Science Daily*, November 7, 2012. https://tinyurl.com/pataabam.

75 Els Adriaens and Jean Paul Remon, "Mucosal Irritation Potential of Personal Lubricants Relates to Product Osmolality as Detected by the Slug Mucosal Irritation Assay," *Sexually Transmitted Diseases* 35:5 (May 2008), 512–16. doi:10.1097/OLQ.0b013e3181644669.

76 Isabelle Gauthier, Lisa Vinebaum, and Rachel Guay, *Hot Pants: Do-It-Yourself Gynecology and Herbal Remedies* (Montreal: Hot Pantz, 1998), 12.

77 Adriaens and Remon, "Mucosal Irritation Potential."

78 K. Kasiram, Prashant Sakharkar, and A. T. Patil, "Antifungal Activity of *Calendula officinalis*," *Indian Journal of Pharmaceutical Sciences.* November–December 2000. https://tinyurl.com/jmns6r7a.

79 Yousef Rahmani et al., "Effect of Herbal Medicine on Vaginal Epithelial Cells: A Systematic Review and Meta-Analysis," *Journal of Menopausal Medicine* 24:1 (April 2018), 11–16. doi:10.6118/jmm.2018.24.1.11.

80 Ibid.

81 Sisi Xi et al., "Effect of Isopropanolic *Cimicifuga racemosa* Extract on Uterine Fibroids in Comparison with Tibolone among Patients of a Recent Randomized, Double Blind, Parallel-Controlled Study in Chinese Women with Menopausal Symptoms," *Complementary and Alternative Medicine* 2014:717686. doi:10.1155/2014/717686.

82 K. Jiang et al., "Black Cohosh Improves Objective Sleep in Postmenopausal Women with Sleep Disturbance," *Climacteric* 18:4 (2015), 559–67. doi:10.3109/13697137.2015.1042450.

83 Heidi Fritz et al., "Black Cohosh and Breast Cancer: A Systematic Review," *Integrative Cancer Therapies* 13:1 (January 2014), 12–29. doi:10.1177/1534735413477191.

84 Rozita Naseri et al., "Comparison of *Vitex agnus-castus* Extracts with Placebo in Reducing Menopausal Symptoms: A Randomized Double-Blind Study," *Korean Journal of Family Medicine* 40:6 (November 2019), 362–67. doi:10.4082/kjfm.18.0067.

85   Margaret Diana van Die et al., "*Vitex agnus-castus* (Chaste-Tree/Berry) in the Treatment of Menopause-Related Complaints," *Journal of Alternative and Complementary Medicine* 15:8 (August 2009), 853–62. doi:10.1089/acm.2008.0447.

86   C. Kupfersztain et al., "The Immediate Effect of Natural Plant Extract, *Angelica sinensis* and *Matricaria chamomilla* (Climex) for the Treatment of Hot Flushes during Menopause: A Preliminary Report," *Clinical and Experimental Obstetrics & Gynecology* 30:4 (2003), 203–6. https://tinyurl.com/bcxrwamn.

87   Carmela Rotem and Boris Kaplan, "Phyto-Female Complex for the Relief of Hot Flushes, Night Sweats and Quality of Sleep: Randomized, Controlled, Double-Blind Pilot Study," *Gynecological Endocrinology* 23:2 (February 2007), 117–22. doi:10.1080/09513590701200900.

88   H. O. Meissner et al., "Use of Gelatinized Maca *(Lepidium peruvianum)* in Early Postmenopausal Women," *International Journal of Biomedical Science* 1:1 (June 2005), 33–45. https://tinyurl.com/tpx38pah.

89   Nicole A. Brooks et al., "Beneficial Effects of *Lepidium meyenii* (Maca) on Psychological Symptoms and Measures of Sexual Dysfunction in Postmenopausal Women Are Not Related to Estrogen or Androgen Content," *Menopause* 15:6 (December 2008), 1157–62. doi:10.1097/gme.0b013e3181732953.

90   Fereshteh Dadfar and Kourosh Bamdad, "The Effect of *Saliva officinalis* Extract on the Menopausal Symptoms in Postmenopausal Women: An RCT," *International Journal of Reproductive Biomedicine* 17:4 (April 2019), 287–92. doi:10.18502/ijrm.v17i4.4555.

91   S. Bommer, P. Klein, and A. Suter, "First-Time Proof of Sage's Tolerability and Efficacy in Menopausal Women with Hot Flushes," *Advances in Therapy* 28:6 (June 2011), 490–500. doi:10.1007/s12325-011-0027-z.

92   Women's Voices for the Earth, "Always Pads Testing Results," n.d. https://tinyurl.com/4wuvsapc.

93   Chan Jin Park et al., "Sanitary Pads and Diapers Contain Higher Phthalate Contents Than Those in Common Commercial Plastic Products," *Reproductive Toxicology* 84 (March 2019), 114–21. doi:10.1016/j.reprotox.2019.01.005.

94   Ulrich Mengs, Ralf-Torsten Pohl, and Todd Mitchell, "The Antidote of Choice in Patients with Acute Hepatotoxicity from Amatoxin Poisoning," *Current Pharmaceutical Biotechnology* 13:10 (August 2012), 1964–70. doi:10.2174/138920112802273353.

95   Tetsuya Akaishi et al., "Successful Treatment of Intractable Menstrual Migraine with the Traditional Herbal Medicine Tokishakuyakusan," *Journal of General and Family Medicine* 20:3 (May 2019), 118–21. doi:10.1002/jgf2.242.

96 Jing-Shu Zhang et al., "Long-Term Exposure to Ambient Air Pollution and Metabolic Syndrome in Children and Adolescents: A National Cross-sectional Study in China," *Environment International* 148 (March 2021). doi:10.1016/j.envint .2021.106383.

97 Jillian Stansbury, "Botanical Influences on Metabolic Syndrome," presentation, American Herbalists Guild, n.d. https://tinyurl.com/nup7cffk.

98 Lawrence Engmann et al., "Racial and Ethnic Differences in the Polycystic Ovary Syndrome (PCOS) Metabolic Phenotype," *American Journal of Obstetrics and Gynecology* 216:5 (May 2017), 493.e1–13. doi:10.1016/j.ajog.2017.01.003.

99 Jennifer K. Hillman et al., "Black Women with Polycystic Ovary Syndrome (PCOS) Have Increased Risk for Metabolic Syndrome and Cardiovascular Disease Compared with White Women with PCOS," *Sexuality, Reproduction & Menopause* 101:2 (February 2014), 530–35. doi:10.1016 /j.fertnstert.2013.10.055.

100 Chan-Young Kwon, Ik-Hyun Cho, and Kyoung Sun Park, "Therapeutic Effects and Mechanisms of Herbal Medicines for Treating Polycystic Ovary Syndrome: A Review," *Frontiers in Pharmacology,* August 12, 2020. doi:10.3389/fphar .2020.01192.

101 Susan Arentz et al., "Herbal Medicine for the Management of Polycystic Ovary Syndrome (PCOS) and Associated Oligo/Amenorrhoea and Hyperandrogenism: A Review of the Laboratory Evidence for Effects with Corroborative Clinical Findings," *BMC Complementary and Alternative Medicine* 14:511 (2014). doi:10.1186/1472-6882-14-511.

102 Jillian Stansbury, "Melissa and Other Dopaminergic Herbs Useful in Treatment of PCOS," *Naturopathic Doctor News and Review,* August 6, 2009. https:// tinyurl.com/rzpk5xy.

103 Arentz et al., "Herbal Medicine."

104 Ibid.

105 Mariann Garner-Wizard et al., "Black Cohosh Stimulates Ovulation Induction in Women with Polycystic Ovarian Syndrome (PCOS)," *HerbClip* 479 (August 30, 2019). https://tinyurl.com/wrk2rr43.

106 Tisheeka Graham-Steed et al., "'Race' and Prostate Cancer Mortality in Equal-access Health Care Systems," *American Journal of Medicine* 126:12 (December 2013), 1084–88. doi:10.1016/j.amjmed.2013.08.012.

107 L. Konrad et al., "Antiproliferative Effect on Human Prostate Cancer Cells by a Stinging Nettle Root *(Urtica dioica)* Extract," *Planta Medica* 66:1 (February 2000), 44–47. doi:10.1055/s-2000-11117.

108 Christopher Nguyen et al., "Dandelion Root and Lemongrass Extracts Induce Apoptosis, Enhance Chemotherapeutic Efficacy, and Reduce Tumour Xeno-graft Growth In Vivo in Prostate Cancer," *Complementary and Alternative Medicine* 2019:2951428. doi:10.1155/2019/2951428.

109 Renea A. Jarred et al., "Induction of Apoptosis in Low to Moderate-Grade Human Prostate Carcinoma by Red Clover-Derived Dietary Isoflavones," *Cancer Epidemiology, Biomarkers & Prevention* 11:12 (2003), 1689–96. https://tinyurl.com/zzn4tyy9.

110 Michael G. Potroz and Nam-Joon Cho, "Natural Products for the Treatment of Trachoma and *Chlamydia trachomatis*," *Molecules* 20:3 (March 2015), 4180–203. doi:10.3390/molecules20034180.

111 N. Vynograd, I. Vynograd, and Z. Sosnowski, "A Comparative Multi-Centre Study of the Efficacy of Propolis, Acyclovir and Placebo in the Treatment of Genital Herpes (HSV)," *Phytomedicine* 7:1 (March 2000), 1–6. doi:10.1016/S0944-7113(00)80014-8.

112 Ayse Yildirim et al., "Antiviral Activity of Hatay Propolis Against Replication of Herpes Simplex Virus Type 1 and Type 2," *Medical Science Monitor* 22 (2016), 422–30. doi:10.12659/MSM.897282.

113 Eric Yarnell, "Herbs Against Human Papillomavirus," *Alternative and Complementary Therapies* 21:2 (April 2015), 71–76. doi:10.1089/act.2015.21205.

114 Dima A. Youssef et al., "The Possible Roles of Vitamin D and Curcumin in Treating Gonorrhea," *Medical Hypotheses* 81:1 (July 2013), 131–35. doi:10.1016/j.mehy.2013.04.013.

115 Sarita Das, "Natural Therapeutics for Urinary Tract Infections—a Review," *Future Journal of Pharmaceutical Sciences* 6:1 (2020), 64. doi:10.1186/s43094-020-00086-2.

116 Bibi Sedigheh Fazly Bazzaz et al., "Deep Insights into Urinary Tract Infections and Effective Natural Remedies," *African Journal of Urology* 27:6 (2021). doi:10.1186/s12301-020-00111-z.

117 Das, "Natural Therapeutics."

118 Zahra Pazhohideh et al., "The Effect of *Calendula officinalis* versus Metronidazole on Bacterial Vaginosis in Women: A Double-Blind Randomized Controlled Trial," *Journal of Advanced Pharmaceutical Technology & Research* 9:1 (January–March 2018), 15–19. doi:10.4103/japtr.JAPTR_305_17.

119 Xiuzhen Ma et al., "Berberine Exhibits Antioxidative Effects and Reduces Apoptosis of the Vaginal Epithelium in Bacterial Vaginosis," *Experimental and Therapeutic Medicine* 18:3 (September 2019), 2122–30. doi:10.3892/etm.2019.7772.

7. Intimate Herbal Materia Medica

1 Mohammad Kaleem Ahmad et al., "*Withania somnifera* Improves Semen Quality by Regulating Reproductive Hormone Levels and Oxidative Stress in Seminal Plasma of Infertile Males," *Fertility and Sterility* 94:3 (August 1, 2010), 989–96. doi:10.1016/j.fertnstert.2009.04.046.

2 Chandrasekhar et al., "Prospective, Randomized Double-Blind, Placebo-Controlled Study."

3 Andrew B. Scholey et al., "Consumption of Cocoa Flavanols Results in Acute Improvements in Mood and Cognitive Performance during Sustained Mental Effort," *Journal of Psychopharmacology* 24:10 (October 2010), 1505–14. doi:10.1177/0269881109106923.

4 Ahmed Al Sunni and Rabia Latif, "Effects of Chocolate Intake on Perceived Stress: A Controlled Clinical Study," *International Journal of Health Sciences, Qassim University* 8:4 (October 2014), 393–401. https://tinyurl.com/3c2fkfx7.

5 Pamela J. Mink et al., "Flavonoid Intake and Cardiovascular Disease Mortality: A Prospective Study in Postmenopausal Women," *American Journal of Clinical Nutrition* 85:3 (March 2007), 895–909. doi:10.1093/ajcn/85.3.895.

6 Brian Buijsse et al., "Cocoa Intake, Blood Pressure, and Cardiovascular Mortality: The Zutphen Elderly Study," *Archives of Internal Medicine* 166:4 (February 27, 2006), 411–17. doi:10.1001/archinte.166.4.411.

7 Pazhohideh et al., "Effect of *Calendula officinalis*."

8 Elnaz Saffari et al., "Comparing the Effects of *Calendula officinalis* and Clotrimazole on Vaginal Candidiasis: A Randomized Controlled Trial," *Women and Health* 57:10 (November–December 2017), 1145–60. doi:10.1080/03630242.2016.1263272.

9 María del Carmen Ramírez Olvera, "Composition of Plant Extracts That Increase Döderlein Bacilli, Used for the Treatment of Sexually Transmitted Diseases (STD) and the Human Papillomavirus (HPV), Having an Aphrodisiac Effect," patent by María del Carmen Ramírez Olvera, filed October 11; 2016, application granted August 6, 2018. https://tinyurl.com/7p33t7am.

10 R. DiPasquale, "Effective Use of Herbal Medicine in Urinary Tract Infections," *Journal of Dietary Supplements* 5:3 (January 1, 2008), 219–28. doi:10.1080/19390210802414220.

11 Atmaca et al., "Effects of *Galium aparine*."

12 Thomas Y. Ito et al., "The Enhancement of Female Sexual Function with ArginMax, a Nutritional Supplement, among Women Differing in

Menopausal Status," *Journal of Sex and Marital Therapy* 32:5 (October–December 2006), 369–78. doi:10.1080/00926230600834901.

13 S. Kumar, R. Madaan, and A. Sharma, "Pharmacological Evaluation of Bioactive Principle of *Turnera aphrodisiaca*," *Indian Journal of Pharmaceutical Sciences* 70:6 (November–December 2008), 740–44. doi:10.4103/0250-474X.49095.

14 "Dandelions (Pu Gong Ying) in Chinese Medicine," Me & Qi, n.d. www.meandqi.com/herb-database/dandelions.

15 Lee Hullender Rubin, Dara Cantor, and Benjamin L. Marx, "Recurrent Pregnancy Loss and Traditional Chinese Medicine," *Medical Acupuncture* 25:3 (June 2013), 232–37. doi:10.1089/acu.2012.0911.

16 Xu Zhi et al., "Dandelion T-1 Extract Up-Regulates Reproductive Hormone Receptor Expression in Mice," *International Journal of Molecular Medicine* 20:3 (September 2007), 287–92. https://pubmed.ncbi.nlm.nih.gov/17671731.

17 Tong Wang et al., "Effect of Dandelion Extracts on the Proliferation of Ovarian Granulosa Cells and Expression of Hormone Receptors," *Chinese Medical Journal* 131:14 (July 20, 2018), 1694–1701. doi:10.4103/0366-6999.235864.

18 Native American Ethnobotany DB, s.v. "taraxacum officinal." https://tinyurl.com/5bcndett.

19 Giti Ozgoli, Marjan Goli, and Fariborz Moattar, "Comparison of Effects of Ginger, Mefenamic Acid, and Ibuprofen on Pain in Women with Primary Dysmenorrhea," *Journal of Alternative and Complementary Medicine* 15:2 (February 2009), 129–32. doi:10.1089/acm.2008.0311.

20 Waleed Abid Al-Kadir Mares and Wisam S. Najam, "The Effect of Ginger on Semen Parameters and Serum FSH, LH & Testosterone of Infertile Men," *Medical Journal of Tikrit University* 18:182 (2012), 322–29. https://tinyurl.com/5y5vxnhb.

21 Mary C. Tassell et al., "Hawthorn (*Crataegus* spp.) in the Treatment of Cardiovascular Disease," *Pharmacognosy Reviews* 4:7 (January–June 2010), 32–41. doi:10.4103/0973-7847.65324.

22 Gustavo F. Gonzales, "Ethnobiology and Ethnopharmacology of *Lepidium meyenii* (Maca), a Plant from the Peruvian Highlands," *Complementary and Alternative Medicine* 2012:193496. doi:10.1155/2012/193496.

23 Gustavo F. Gonzales et al., "Effect of *Lepidium meyenii* (Maca) on Sexual Desire and Its Absent Relationship with Serum Testosterone Levels in Adult Healthy Men," *Andrologia* 34:6 (December 2002), 367–72. doi:10.1046/j.1439-0272.2002.00519.x.

24 Christina M. Dording et al., "A Double-Blind Placebo-Controlled Trial of Maca Root as Treatment for Antidepressant-Induced Sexual Dysfunction in Women," *Complementary and Alternative Medicine* 2015:949036. doi:10.1155/2015/949036.

25 Gonzales, "Ethnobiology and Ethnopharmacology."

26 Kanitta Jiraungkoorskul and Wannee Jiraungkoorskul, "Review of Naturopathy of Medical Mushroom, Ophiocordyceps Sinensis, in Sexual Dysfunction," *Pharmacognosy Reviews* 10:19 (January–June 2016), 1–5. doi:10.4103/0973 -7847.176566.

27 Tito Fernandes, Eusébio Chaquisse, and Jorge Ferrão, "HIV and the Antiviral Role of Mushroom Nutraceuticals," *European Journal of Applied Sciences* 8:3 (2020). doi:10.14738/aivp.83.8650.

28 Alireza Ghorbanibirgani, Ali Khalili, and Laleh Zamani, "The Efficacy of Stinging Nettle *(Urtica dioica)* in Patients with Benign Prostatic Hyperplasia: A Randomized Double-Blind Study in 100 Patients," *Iranian Red Crescent Medical Journal* 15:1 (January 2013), 9–10. doi:10.5812/ircmj.2386.

29 Gayle Engels and Josef Brinckmann, "Stinging Nettle," *HerbalGram* 110 (Summer 2016), 8–16. https://tinyurl.com/nzpjmpmm.

30 David O. Kennedy et al., "Acute and Chronic Effects of Green Oat *(Avena sativa)* Extract on Cognitive Function and Mood during a Laboratory Stressor in Healthy Adults: A Randomized, Double-Blind, Placebo-Controlled Study in Healthy Humans," *Nutrients* 12:6 (June 2020), 1598. doi:10.3390/nu12061598.

31 Neelesh Malviya et al., "Recent Studies on Aphrodisiac Herbs for the Management of Male Sexual Dysfunction—a Review," *Acta Poloniae Pharmaceutica* 68:1 (January–February 2011), 3–8. https://tinyurl.com/ux4cvy33.

32 M. Akdoğan et al., "The Effects of Milled *Tribulus terrestris, Avena sativa,* and White Ginseng Powder on Total Cholesterol, Free Testosterone Levels and Testicular Tissue in Rats Fed a High-Cholesterol Diet," *Veteriner Fakültesi dergisi* 65:3 (January 2018), 267–72. doi:10.1501/Vetfak_0000002856.

33 Lara Pacheco, "Oats *(Avena sativa),*" HerbRally, n.d. www.herbrally.com /monographs/oats.

34 M. Ghazanfarpour et al., "Red Clover for Treatment of Hot Flashes and Menopausal Symptoms: A Systematic Review and Meta-Analysis," *Journal of Obstetrics and Gynaecology* 36:3 (2016), 301–11. doi:10.3109/01443615.2015.1049249.

35 Pragya Gartoulla and Myo Mint Han, "Red Clover Extract for Alleviating Hot Flushes in Postmenopausal Women: A Meta-Analysis," *Maturitas* 79:1 (September 2014), 58–64. doi:10.1016/j.maturitas.2014.06.018.

36 Bunce, "Herbs and Somatic Practices."

37 Ying-Fen Tseng, Chung-Hey Chen, and Yi-Hsin Yang, "Rose Tea for Relief of Primary Dysmenorrhea in Adolescents: A Randomized Controlled Trial in Taiwan," *Journal of Midwifery & Women's Health* 50:5 (September–October 2005), e51–57. doi:10.1016/j.jmwh.2005.06.003.

38 S. K. Jin and J. H. Park, "Effect of the Addition of *Schisandra chinensis* Powder on the Physico-chemical Characteristics of Sausage," *Asian-Australasian Journal of Animal Sciences* 26:12 (December 2013), 1753–61. doi:10.5713/ajas.2013.13194.

39 Jane Teas et al., "The Consumption of Seaweed as a Protective Factor in the Etiology of Breast Cancer: Proof of Principle," *Journal of Applied Phycology* 25:3 (2013), 771–79. doi:10.1007/s10811-012-9931-0.

40 Anderson Fellyp Avelino Diniz et al., "Potential Therapeutic Role of Dietary Supplementation with *Spirulina platensis* on the Erectile Function of Obese Rats Fed a Hypercaloric Diet," *Oxidative Medicine and Cellular Longevity* 2020:3293065. doi:10.1155/2020/3293065.

41 Dae Yeon Cho et al., "Studies on the Biosorption of Heavy Metals onto *Chlorella vulgaris*," *Journal of Environmental Science and Health A* 29:2 (December 2008), 389–409. doi:10.1080/10934529409376043.

42 Feng Guo et al., "Dietary Seaweed Intake and Depressive Symptoms in Japanese Adults: A Prospective Cohort Study," *Nutrition Journal* 18:58 (2019). doi:10.1186/s12937-019-0486-7.

43 Jairam Meena et al., "*Asparagus racemosus* Competitively Inhibits In Vitro the Acetylcholine and Monoamine Metabolizing Enzymes," *Neuroscience Letters* 503:1 (September 26, 2011), 6–9. doi:10.1016/j.neulet.2011.07.051.

44 D. Bhattacharyya et al., "Controlled Programmed Trial of *Ocimum sanctum* Leaf on Generalized Anxiety Disorders," *Nepal Medical College Journal* 10:3 (September 2008), 176–79. https://tinyurl.com/5jxefyar.

45 Ram Chandra Saxena et al., "Efficacy of an Extract of *Ocimum tenuiflorum* (OciBest) in the Management of General Stress: A Double-Blind, Placebo-Controlled Study," *Complementary and Alternative Medicine* 2012:894509. doi:10.1155/2012/894509.

46 Claudia Daniele et al., "*Vitex agnus-castus*: A Systematic Review of Adverse Events," *Drug Safety* 28 (2005), 319–32. doi:10.2165/00002018-200528040-00004.

47 Mikio Momoeda et al., "Efficacy and Safety of *Vitex agnus-castus* Extract for Treatment of Premenstrual Syndrome in Japanese Patients: A Prospective, Open-Label Study," *Advances in Therapy* 31:3 (March 2014), 362–73. doi:10.1007/s12325-014-0106-z.

48 Lynn M. Westphal et al., "A Nutritional Supplement for Improving Fertility in Women: A Pilot Study," *Journal of Reproductive Medicine* 49:4 (April 2004), 289–93. https://tinyurl.com/p34vaf54.

49 Naseri et al., "Comparison of *Vitex agnus-castus.*"

Bibliography

Abascal, Kathy, and Eric Yarnell. "Botanical Treatments for Hemorrhoids." *Alternative and Complementary Therapies* 11:6 (December 2005), 285–89. doi:10.1089/act.2005.11.285.

Abdel-Wahhab, Khaled G., Hagar H. Mourad, Fathia A. Mannaa, Fatma A. Morsy, Laila K. Hassan, and Rehab F. Taher. "Role of Ashwagandha Methanolic Extract in the Regulation of Thyroid Profile in Hypothyroidism Modeled Rats." *Molecular Biology Reports* 46 (2019), 3637–49. doi:10.1007/s11033-019-04721-x.

Aboelsoud, N. H. "Herbal Medicine in Ancient Egypt." *Journal of Medicinal Plants Research* 4:2 (December 8, 2009), 82–86. doi:10.5897/JMPR09.013.

Abubakar, Abdullahi R., and Mainul Haque. "Preparation of Medicinal Plants: Basic Extraction and Fractionation Procedures for Experimental Purposes." *Journal of Pharmacy and Bioallied Sciences* 12:1 (January–March 2020), 1–10. doi:10.4103/jpbs.JPBS_175_19.

Adriaens, Els, and Jean Paul Remon. "Mucosal Irritation Potential of Personal Lubricants Relates to Product Osmolality as Detected by the Slug Mucosal Irritation Assay." *Sexually Transmitted Diseases* 35:5 (May 2008), 512–16. doi:10.1097/OLQ.0b013e3181644669.

Ahmad, Mohammad Kaleem, Abbas Ali Mahdi, Kamla Kant Shukla, Najmul Islam, Singh Rajender, Dama Madhukar, Satya Narain Shankhwar, and Sohail Ahmad. "*Withania somnifera* Improves Semen Quality by Regulating Reproductive Hormone Levels and Oxidative Stress in Seminal Plasma of Infertile Males." *Fertility and Sterility* 94:3 (August 1, 2010), 989–96. doi:10.1016/j.fertnstert.2009.04.046.

Ainehchi, Nava, Arash Khaki, Azizeh Farshbaf-Khalili, Mohamad Hammadeh, and Elaheh Ouladsahebmadarek. "The Effectiveness of Herbal Mixture Supplements with and without Clomiphene Citrate in Comparison to Clomiphene Citrate on Serum Antioxidants and Glycemic Biomarkers in Women with Polycystic Ovary Syndrome Willing to Be Pregnant: A Randomized Clinical Trial." *Biomolecules* 9:6 (June 2019), 215. doi:10.3390/biom9060215.

Akaishi, Tetsuya, Shin Takayama, Minoru Ohsawa, Akiko Kikuchi, Ryutaro Arita, Ichiro Nakashima, Masashi Aoki, and Tadashi Ishii. "Successful Treatment of Intractable Menstrual Migraine with the Traditional Herbal Medicine Toki-shakuyakusan." *Journal of General and Family Medicine* 20:3 (May 2019), 118–21. doi:10.1002/jgf2.242.

Akdoğan, M., Y. Nasir, N. Cengiz, and A. Bilgili. "The Effects of Milled *Tribulus terrestris, Avena sativa,* and White Ginseng Powder on Total Cholesterol, Free Testosterone Levels and Testicular Tissue in Rats Fed a High-Cholesterol Diet." *Veteriner Fakültesi dergisi* 65:3 (January 2018), 267–72. doi:10.1501 /Vetfak_0000002856.

Al Sunni, Ahmed, and Rabia Latif. "Effects of Chocolate Intake on Perceived Stress: A Controlled Clinical Study." *International Journal of Health Sciences, Qassim University* 8:4 (October 2014), 393–401. https://tinyurl.com/3c2fkfx7.

Alipanah, Hiva, Mohammad Reza Bigdeli, and Mohammad Ali Esmaeili. "Inhibitory Effect of *Viola odorata* Extract on Tumor Growth and Metastasis in 4T1 Breast Cancer Model." *Iranian Journal of Pharmaceutical Research* 17:1 (Winter 2018), 276–91. https://tinyurl.com/3u4pbskn.

American Psychological Association. "Stress Effects on the Body." November 1, 2018. www.apa.org/topics/stress/body.

Arentz, Susan, Jason Anthony Abbott, Caroline Anne Smith, and Alan Bensoussan. "Herbal Medicine for the Management of Polycystic Ovary Syndrome (PCOS) and Associated Oligo/Amenorrhoea and Hyperandrogenism: A Review of the Laboratory Evidence for Effects with Corroborative Clinical Findings." *BMC Complementary and Alternative Medicine* 14:511 (2014). doi:10.1186/1472-6882-14-511.

Arvigo, Rosita. "My Mentors." November 9, 2020. https://rositaarvigo.com/about /my-mentors.

Atkinson, Charlotte, Ruth M. L. Warren, Evis Sala, Mitch Dowsett, Alison M. Dunning, Catherine S. Healey, Shirley Runswick, Nicholas E. Day, and Sheila A. Bingham. "Red Clover–Derived Isoflavones and Mammographic Breast Density: A Double-Blind, Randomized, Placebo-Controlled Trial." *Breast Cancer Research* 6:R170–79 (February 24, 2004). doi:10.1186/bcr773.

Atmaca, Harika, Emir Bozkurt, Mustafa Cittan, and Hafize Dilek Tepe. "Effects of *Galium aparine* Extract on the Cell Viability, Cell Cycle and Cell Death in Breast Cancer Cell Lines." *Journal of Ethnopharmacology* 186 (June 20, 2016), 305–10. doi:10.1016/j.jep.2016.04.007.

Bae, In Young, Bo-Yeon Kwak, and Hyeon Gyu Lee. "Synergistic Antiradical Action of Natural Antioxidants and Herbal Mixture for Preventing Dioxin Toxicity." *Food Science and Biotechnology* 21 (2012), 491–96. doi:10.1007/s10068-012-0062-9.

Balick, Michael J., and Hugh O'Brien. "Ethnobotanical and Floristic Research in Belize: Accomplishments, Challenges and Lessons Learned." *Ethnobotany Research and Applications* 2 (2004), 77–88. https://tinyurl.com/3knmrze9.

Bazzaz, Bibi Sedigheh Fazly, Sareh Darvishi Fork, Reza Ahmadi, and Bahman Khameneh. "Deep Insights into Urinary Tract Infections and Effective Natural Remedies." *African Journal of Urology* 27:6 (2021). doi:10.1186/s12301-020-00111-z.

Beck, V., U. Rohr, and A. Jungbauer. "Phytoestrogens Derived from Red Clover: An Alternative to Estrogen Replacement Therapy?" *Journal of Steroid Biochemistry and Molecular Biology* 94:5 (March 23, 2005), 499–518. doi:10.1016/j.jsbmb.2004 .12.038.

Bennett, Robin Rose. "Wild Carrot Exploration." Herbal Medicine and EarthSpirit Teachings. August 2011. https://tinyurl.com/4taafvf9.

Bhattacharyya, D., T. K. Sur, U. Jana, and P. K. Debnath. "Controlled Programmed Trial of *Ocimum sanctum* Leaf on Generalized Anxiety Disorders." *Nepal Medical College Journal* 10:3 (September 2008), 176–79. https://tinyurl.com/5jxefyar.

Birla, Hareram, Chetan Keswani, Sachchida Nand Rai, Saumitra Sen Singh, Walia Zahra, and Hagera Dilnashin. "Neuroprotective Effects of *Withania somnifera* in BPA-Induced Cognitive Dysfunction and Oxidative Stress in Mice." *Behavioral and Brain Functions* 15:1 (May 7, 2019). https://tinyurl.com/8h2zmk5c.

Biswal, Biswa Mohan, Siti Amrah Sulaiman, Hasanah Che Ismail, Hasmat Zakaria, and Kamarul Imran Musa. "Effect of *Withania somnifera* (Ashwagandha) on the Development of Chemotherapy-Induced Fatigue and Quality of Life in Breast Cancer Patients." *Integrative Cancer Therapies* 12:4 (July 2013), 312–22. doi:10.1177/1534735412464551.

Bommer, S., P. Klein, and A. Suter. "First-Time Proof of Sage's Tolerability and Efficacy in Menopausal Women with Hot Flushes." *Advances in Therapy* 28:6 (June 2011), 490–500. doi:10.1007/s12325-011-0027-z.

Borrell-Carrió, Francesc, Anthony L. Suchman, and Ronald M. Epstein. "The Biopsychosocial Model 25 Years Later: Principles, Practice, and Scientific Inquiry." *Annals of Family Medicine* 2:6 (2004), 576–82. doi:10.1370/afm.245.

Brooks, Nicole A., Gisela Wilcox, Karen Z. Walker, John F. Ashton, Marc B. Cox, and Lily Stojanovska. "Beneficial Effects of *Lepidium meyenii* (Maca) on Psychological Symptoms and Measures of Sexual Dysfunction in Postmenopausal

Women Are Not Related to Estrogen or Androgen Content." *Menopause* 15:6 (December 2008), 1157–62. doi:10.1097/gme.0b013e3181732953.

Brower, Vicki. "Mind-body Research Moves Towards the Mainstream." *European Molecular Biology Organization Reports* 7:4 (2006), 358–61. doi:10.1038/sj.embor .7400671.

Brown, E. Richard. *Rockefeller Medicine Men: Medicine and Capitalism in America.* Berkeley, CA: University of California Press, 1979.

Buijsse, Brian, Edith J. M. Feskens, Frans J. Kok, and Daan Kromhout. "Cocoa Intake, Blood Pressure, and Cardiovascular Mortality: The Zutphen Elderly Study." *Archives of Internal Medicine* 166:4 (February 27, 2006), 411–17. doi:10.1001 /archinte.166.4.411.

Bunce, Larken. "Herbs and Somatic Practices for Stress, Trauma and Resilience." Dandelion Seed Conference, Olympia, WA, 2017. https://tinyurl.com/42ephxtj.

Cao, Huijuan, Mei Han, Ernest H. Y. Ng, Xiaoke Wu, Andrew Flower, George Lewith, and Jian-Ping Liu. "Can Chinese Herbal Medicine Improve Outcomes of In Vitro Fertilization? A Systematic Review and Meta-Analysis of Randomized Controlled Trials." *PLoS One* 8:12 (2013), e81650. doi:10.1371/journal.pone.0081650.

Capogrosso, Paolo, Michele Colicchia, Eugenio Ventimiglia, Giulia Castagna, Maria Chiara Clementi, Nazareno Suardi, Fabio Castiglione, et al. "One Patient Out of Four with Newly Diagnosed Erectile Dysfunction Is a Young Man—Worrisome Picture from the Everyday Clinical Practice." *Journal of Sexual Medicine* 10:7 (2013). doi:10.1111/jsm.12179.

Casado-Espada, Nerea M., Rubén de Alarcón, Javier I. de la Iglesia-Larrad, Berta Bote-Bonaechea, and Ángel L. Montejo. "Hormonal Contraceptives, Female Sexual Dysfunction, and Managing Strategies: A Review." *Journal of Clinical Medicine* 8:6 (June 2019), 908. doi:10.3390/jcm8060908.

Chandrasekhar, K., Jyoti Kapoor, and Sridhar Anishetty. "A Prospective, Randomized Double-Blind, Placebo-Controlled Study of Safety and Efficacy of a High-Concentration Full-Spectrum Extract of Ashwagandha Root in Reducing Stress and Anxiety in Adults." *Indian Journal of Psychological Medicine* 34:3 (July–September 2012), 255–62. doi:10.4103/0253-7176.106022.

Chauhan, Nagendra Singh, Vikas Sharma, V. K. Dixit, and Mayank Thakur. "A Review on Plants Used for Improvement of Sexual Performance and Virility." *Biomed Research International* 2014 (August 18, 2014). doi:10.1155/2014/868062.

Cho, Dae Yeon, Sung Taik Lee, Sang Won Park, and An Sik Chung. "Studies on the Biosorption of Heavy Metals onto *Chlorella vulgaris*." *Journal of*

Environmental Science and Health A 29:2 (December 2008), 389–409. doi: 10.1080/10934529409376043.

Cohen, A. J., and B. Bartlik. "*Ginkgo biloba* for Antidepressant-Induced Sexual Dysfunction." *Journal of Sex and Marital Therapy* 24:2 (April–June 1998), 139–43. doi:10.1080/00926239808404927.

Cole, Bob. "'The Very Future of Our Nations': How Aboriginal Midwifery Represents a Practical Model for Utilization of Traditional Knowledge." *Journal of Integrated Studies* 10:1 (2018). https://tinyurl.com/th9x776r.

Cusatis, Rachel, Nicole Fergestrom, Alexandra Cooper, Kate D. Schoyer, Abbey Kruper, Jay Sandlow, Estil Strawn, and Kathryn E. Flynn. "Too Much Time? Time Use and Fertility-specific Quality of Life among Men and Women Seeking Specialty Care for Infertility." *BMC Psychology* 7:45 (2019). doi:10.1186/s40359 -019-0312-1.

Dadfar, Fereshteh, and Kourosh Bamdad. "The Effect of *Saliva officinalis* Extract on the Menopausal Symptoms in Postmenopausal Women: An RCT." *International Journal of Reproductive Biomedicine* 17:4 (April 2019), 287–92. doi:10.18502 /ijrm.v17i4.4555.

"Dandelions (Pu Gong Ying) in Chinese Medicine." Me & Qi, n.d. www.meandqi .com/herb-database/dandelions.

Daniele, Claudia, Joanna Thompson Coon, Max H. Pittler, and Edzard Ernst. "*Vitex agnus-castus:* A Systematic Review of Adverse Events." *Drug Safety* 28 (2005), 319–32. doi:10.2165/00002018-200528040-00004.

Das, Sarita. "Natural Therapeutics for Urinary Tract Infections—a Review." *Future Journal of Pharmaceutical Sciences* 6:1 (2020), 64. doi:10.1186/s43094 -020-00086-2.

Defarge, N., J. Spiroux de Vendômois, and G. E. Séralini. "Toxicity of Formulants and Heavy Metals in Glyphosate-Based Herbicides and Other Pesticides." *Toxicology Reports* 5 (2018), 156–63. doi:10.1016/j.toxrep.2017.12.025.

Diniz, Anderson Fellyp Avelino, Iara Leão Luna de Souza, Elba dos Santos Ferreira, Maria Thaynan de Lima Carvalho, Bárbara Cavalcanti Barros, Paula Benvindo Ferreira, Maria da Conceição Correia Silva, et al. "Potential Therapeutic Role of Dietary Supplementation with *Spirulina platensis* on the Erectile Function of Obese Rats Fed a Hypercaloric Diet." *Oxidative Medicine and Cellular Longevity* 2020:3293065. doi:10.1155/2020/3293065.

DiPasquale, R. "Effective Use of Herbal Medicine in Urinary Tract Infections." *Journal of Dietary Supplements* 5:3 (January 1, 2008), 219–28. doi:10.1080/19390210802414220.

Dording, Christina M. "Safety and Effectiveness Study of Maca Root to Treat Antidepressant-Induced Sexual Dysfunction." ClinicalTrials.gov. 2019. https://tinyurl.com/utayy3yr.

Dording, Christina M., Pamela J. Schettler, Elizabeth D. Dalton, Susannah R. Parkin, Rosemary S. W. Walker, Kara B. Fehling, Maurizio Fava, and David Mischoulon. "A Double-Blind Placebo-Controlled Trial of Maca Root as Treatment for Antidepressant-Induced Sexual Dysfunction in Women." *Complementary and Alternative Medicine* 2015:949036. doi:10.1155/2015/949036.

Duncan, Sophie. "Critical Relationality: Queer, Indigenous, and Multispecies Belonging Beyond Settler Sex & Nature." *Imaginations,* July 25, 2019. doi:10.17742/IMAGE.CR.10.1.4. https://tinyurl.com/4r5y8x4s.

Dyck, Roland, Nathaniel Osgood, Ting Hsiang Lin, Amy Gao, and Mary Rose Stang. "Epidemiology of Diabetes Mellitus among First Nations and Non–First Nations Adults." *Canadian Medical Association Journal* 182:3 (February 2010), 249–56. doi:10.1503/cmaj.090846.

Engels, Gayle, and Josef Brinckmann. "Stinging Nettle." *HerbalGram* 110 (Summer 2016), 8–16. https://tinyurl.com/nzpjmpmm.

Engmann, Lawrence, Susan Jin, Fangbai Sun, Richard S. Legro, Alex J. Polotsky, Karl R. Hansen, Christos Coutifaris, et al. "Racial and Ethnic Differences in the Polycystic Ovary Syndrome (PCOS) Metabolic Phenotype." *American Journal of Obstetrics and Gynecology* 216:5 (May 2017), 493.e1–13. doi:10.1016/j.ajog.2017.01.003.

European Medicines Agency. "Assessment Report on *Avena sativa* L., Herba and *Avena sativa* L., Fructus." September 4, 2008. https://tinyurl.com/6j645hr7.

Evidence-Based Medicine Consult. "Medication & Herbal Inhibitors of the Cytochrome P450 (CYP) Enzymes Drug Table." n.d. https://tinyurl.com/5xnvsjdb.

Fernandes, Tito, Eusébio Chaquisse, and Jorge Ferrão. "HIV and the Antiviral Role of Mushroom Nutraceuticals." *European Journal of Applied Sciences* 8:3 (2020). doi:10.14738/aivp.83.8650.

Fritz, Heidi, Dugald Seely, Jessie McGowan, Becky Skidmore, Rochelle Fernandes, Deborah A. Kennedy, Kieran Cooley, et al. "Black Cohosh and Breast Cancer: A Systematic Review." *Integrative Cancer Therapies* 13:1 (January 2014), 12–29. doi:10.1177/1534735413477191.

Galimova, E. F., Z. K. Amirova, and S. N. Galimov. "Dioxins in the Semen of Men with Infertility." *Environmental Science and Pollution Research International* 22:19 (October 2015), 14566–69. doi:10.1007/s11356-014-3109-z.

Garner-Wizard, Mariann, Shari Henson, Dani Hoots, Samaara Robbins, and Gavin Van De Walle. "Adjunct Treatment with Ashwagandha Root Extract for Fatigue from Chemotherapy for Breast Cancer." *HerbClip* June 14, 2013. https://tinyurl.com/6cv2zuf4.

Garner-Wizard, Mariann, Shari Henson, Dani Hoots, Samaara Robbins, and Gavin Van De Walle. "Black Cohosh Stimulates Ovulation Induction in Women with Polycystic Ovarian Syndrome (PCOS)." *HerbClip* 479 (August 30, 2019). https://tinyurl.com/wrk2rr43.

Gartoulla, Pragya, and Myo Mint Han. "Red Clover Extract for Alleviating Hot Flushes in Postmenopausal Women: A Meta-Analysis." *Maturitas* 79:1 (September 2014), 58–64. doi:10.1016/j.maturitas.2014.06.018.

Gauthier, Isabelle, Lisa Vinebaum, and Rachel Guay. *Hot Pants: Do-It-Yourself Gynecology and Herbal Remedies.* Montreal: Hot Pantz, 1998.

Ghazanfarpour, M., R. Sadeghi, R. Latifnejad Roudsari, I. Khorsand, T. Khadivzadeh, and B. Muoio. "Red Clover for Treatment of Hot Flashes and Menopausal Symptoms: A Systematic Review and Meta-Analysis." *Journal of Obstetrics and Gynaecology* 36:3 (2016), 301–11. doi:10.3109/01443615.2015.1049249.

Ghorbanibirgani, Alireza, Ali Khalili, and Laleh Zamani. "The Efficacy of Stinging Nettle *(Urtica dioica)* in Patients with Benign Prostatic Hyperplasia: A Randomized Double-Blind Study in 100 Patients." *Iranian Red Crescent Medical Journal* 15:1 (January 2013), 9–10. doi:10.5812/ircmj.2386.

Giuliano, F., and J. Allard. "Dopamine and Sexual Function." *International Journal of Impotence Research* Suppl. 3 (August 13, 2001), S18–28. doi:10.1038/sj.ijir.3900719.

Goldstein, Irwin. "The Central Mechanisms of Sexual Function." Boston University School of Medicine. February 7, 2003. https://tinyurl.com/w4any5bd.

Gonzales, Gustavo F. "Ethnobiology and Ethnopharmacology of *Lepidium meyenii* (Maca), a Plant from the Peruvian Highlands." *Complementary and Alternative Medicine* 2012:193496. doi:10.1155/2012/193496.

Gonzales, Gustavo F., A. Córdova, K. Vega, A. Chung, A. Villena, C. Góñez, and S. Castillo. "Effect of *Lepidium meyenii* (Maca) on Sexual Desire and Its Absent Relationship with Serum Testosterone Levels in Adult Healthy Men." *Andrologia* 34:6 (December 2002), 367–72. doi:10.1046/j.1439-0272.2002.00519.x.

Graham-Steed, Tisheeka, Edward Uchio, Carolyn K. Wells, Mihaela Aslan, John Ko, and John Concato. "'Race' and Prostate Cancer Mortality in Equal-access Health Care Systems." *American Journal of Medicine* 126:12 (December 2013), 1084–88. doi:10.1016/j.amjmed.2013.08.012.

Guo, Feng, Cong Huang, Yufei Cui, Haruki Momma, Kaijun Niu, and Ryoichi Nagatomi. "Dietary Seaweed Intake and Depressive Symptoms in Japanese Adults: A Prospective Cohort Study." *Nutrition Journal* 18:58 (2019). doi:10.1186/s12937-019-0486-7.

Hamilton, Lisa Dawn, Alessandra H. Rellini, and Cindy M. Meston. "Cortisol, Sexual Arousal, and Affect in Response to Sexual Stimuli." *Journal of Sexual Medicine* 5:9 (September 2008), 2111–18. doi:10.1111/j.1743-6109.2008.00922.x.

Higgins, Agnes, Michael Nash, and Aileen M. Lynch. "Antidepressant-Associated Sexual Dysfunction: Impact, Effects, and Treatment." *Drug, Healthcare and Patient Safety* 2 (2010), 141–50. doi:10.2147/DHPS.S7634.

Hillman, Jennifer K., Lauren N. C. Johnson, Meghana Limaye, Rebecca A. Feldman, Mary Sammel, and Anuja Dokras. "Black Women with Polycystic Ovary Syndrome (PCOS) Have Increased Risk for Metabolic Syndrome and Cardiovascular Disease Compared with White Women with PCOS." *Sexuality, Reproduction & Menopause* 101:2 (February 2014), 530–35. doi:10.1016/j.fertnstert.2013.10.055.

Ilhan, Mert, Fatma Tuğçe Gürağaç Dereli, and Esra Küpeli Akkol. "Novel Drug Targets with Traditional Herbal Medicines for Overcoming Endometriosis." *Current Drug Delivery* 16:5 (June 2019), 386–99. doi:10.2174/1567201816666181227112421.

Integrative Herbalism, Summer 2014 issue. Vermont Center for Integrative Herbalism. https://tinyurl.com/4wskv73p.

Ito, Thomas Y., Mary Lake Polan, Beverly Whipple, and Aileen Sontag Trant. "The Enhancement of Female Sexual Function with ArginMax, a Nutritional Supplement, among Women Differing in Menopausal Status." *Journal of Sex and Marital Therapy* 32:5 (October–December 2006), 369–78. doi:10.1080/00926230600834901.

Jarred, Renea A., Mohammad Keikha, Caroline Dowling, Stephen McPherson, Anne Clare, Alan Husband, John Pedersen, Mark Frydenberg, and Gail Risbridger. "Induction of Apoptosis in Low to Moderate-Grade Human Prostate Carcinoma by Red Clover-Derived Dietary Isoflavones." *Cancer Epidemiology, Biomarkers & Prevention* 11:12 (2003), 1689–96. https://tinyurl.com/zzn4tyy9.

Jesse, Caffyn. "Elements of Intimacy: The Dance of Loving Connection." *EroSpirit.* Independently published. July 4, 2019.

Jiang, K., Y. Jin, L. Huang, S. Feng, X. Hou, B. Du, J. Zheng, and L. Li. "Black Cohosh Improves Objective Sleep in Postmenopausal Women with Sleep Disturbance." *Climacteric* 18:4 (2015), 559–67. doi:10.3109/13697137.2015.1042450.

Jin, S. K., and J. H. Park. "Effect of the Addition of *Schisandra chinensis* Powder on the Physico-chemical Characteristics of Sausage." *Asian-Australasian Journal of Animal Sciences* 26:12 (December 2013), 1753–61. doi:10.5713/ajas.2013.13194.

Jiraungkoorskul, Kanitta, and Wannee Jiraungkoorskul. "Review of Naturopathy of Medical Mushroom, Ophiocordyceps Sinensis, in Sexual Dysfunction." *Pharmacognosy Reviews* 10:19 (January–June 2016), 1–5. doi:10.4103/0973-7847 .176566.

Jouhari, Sheyda, Afsaneh Mohammadzadeh, Haleh Soltanghoraee, Zohreh Mohammadi, Shaheen Khazali, Ebrahim Mirzadegan, Niknam Lakpour, et al. "Effects of Silymarin, Cabergoline and Letrozole on Rat Model of Endometriosis." *Taiwanese Journal of Obstetrics and Gynecology* 57:6 (December 2018), 830–35. doi:10.1016/j.tjog.2018.10.011.

Karst, Amanda. "Conservation Value of the North American Boreal Forest from an Ethnobotanical Perspective." Canadian Boreal Initiative, 2010. https:// tinyurl.com/7ed746vu.

Kasiram, K., Prashant Sakharkar, and A. T. Patil. "Antifungal Activity of *Calendula officinalis*." *Indian Journal of Pharmaceutical Sciences*. November–December 2000. https://tinyurl.com/jmns6r7a.

Kennedy, David O., Bernd Bonnländer, Stefanie C. Lang, Ivo Pischel, Joanne Forster, Julie Khan, Philippa A. Jackson, and Emma L. Wightman. "Acute and Chronic Effects of Green Oat *(Avena sativa)* Extract on Cognitive Function and Mood during a Laboratory Stressor in Healthy Adults: A Randomized, Double-Blind, Placebo-Controlled Study in Healthy Humans." *Nutrients* 12:6 (June 2020), 1598. doi:10.3390/nu12061598.

Kessler, Anna, Sam Sollie, Ben Challacombe, Karen Briggs, and Mieke Van Hemelrijck. "The Global Prevalence of Erectile Dysfunction: A Review." *BJU International* 124:4 (October 2019), 587–99. doi:10.1111/bju.14813.

Ki-moon, Park, Hwang Jin-guk, and Kim Hyun-seok. "An Oriental Herb Extracts Composition Having Detoxification Effect on the Nicotine and Dioxin." Patent by Hyunseok Kim. Filed September 5, 2003. Application granted November 8, 2005. https://patents.google.com/patent /KR100526760B1/en.

Kong, Sai, Yue-Hui Zhang, Chen-Fang Liu, Ilene Tsui, Ying Guo, Bei-Bei Ai, and Feng-Juan Han. "The Complementary and Alternative Medicine for Endometriosis: A Review of Utilization and Mechanism." *Complementary and Alternative Medicine* 2014:146383. doi:10.1155/2014/146383.

Konrad, L., H. H. Müller, C. Lenz, H. Laubinger, G. Aumüller, and J. J. Lichius. "Antiproliferative Effect on Human Prostate Cancer Cells by a Stinging Nettle Root *(Urtica dioica)* Extract." *Planta Medica* 66:1 (February 2000), 44–47. doi:10.1055/s-2000-11117.

Koual, Meriem, Céline Tomkiewicz, German Cano-Sancho, Jean-Philippe Antignac, Anne-Sophie Bats, and Xavier Coumoul. "Environmental Chemicals, Breast Cancer Progression and Drug Resistance." *Environmental Health* 19:117 (2020). doi:10.1186/s12940-020-00670-2.

Kumar, S., R. Madaan, and A. Sharma. "Pharmacological Evaluation of Bioactive Principle of *Turnera aphrodisiaca*." *Indian Journal of Pharmaceutical Sciences* 70:6 (November–December 2008), 740–44. doi:10.4103/0250-474X.49095.

Kupfersztain, C., C. Rotem, R. Fagot, and B. Kaplan. "The Immediate Effect of Natural Plant Extract, *Angelica sinensis* and *Matricaria chamomilla* (Climex) for the Treatment of Hot Flushes during Menopause: A Preliminary Report." *Clinical and Experimental Obstetrics & Gynecology* 30:4 (2003), 203–6. https://tinyurl.com/bcxrwamn.

Kwon, Chan-Young, Ik-Hyun Cho, and Kyoung Sun Park. "Therapeutic Effects and Mechanisms of Herbal Medicines for Treating Polycystic Ovary Syndrome: A Review." *Frontiers in Pharmacology,* August 12, 2020. doi:10.3389/fphar.2020.01192.

Laganà, Antonio Simone, Valentina Lucia La Rosa, Agnese Maria Chiara Rapisarda, Gaetano Valenti, Fabrizio Sapia, Benito Chiofalo, Diego Rossetti, Helena Ban Frangež, Eda Vrtačnik Bokal, and Salvatore Giovanni Vitale. "Anxiety and Depression in Patients with Endometriosis: Impact and Management Challenges." *International Journal of Women's Health* 9 (2017), 323–30. doi:10.2147/IJWH.S119729.

Lee, Hye Won, Myeong Soo Lee, Tae Hun Kim, Terje Alraek, Chris Zaslawski, Jong Wook Kim, and Du Geon Moon. "Ginseng for Erectile Dysfunction." *Cochrane Database of Systematic Reviews* 2017:5 (May 2017), CD012654. doi:10.1002/14651858.CD012654.

Liao, Guo-Shiou, Maria Karmella Apaya, and Lie-Fen Shyur. "Herbal Medicine and Acupuncture for Breast Cancer Palliative Care and Adjuvant Therapy." *Complementary and Alternative Medicine* 2013:437948. doi:10.1155/2013/437948.

Lopresti, Adrian L., Peter D. Drummond, and Stephen J. Smith. "A Randomized, Double-Blind, Placebo-Controlled, Crossover Study Examining the Hormonal and Vitality Effects of Ashwagandha *(Withania somnifera)* in Aging, Overweight Males." *American Journal of Men's Health* 13:2 (March–April 2019). doi:10.1177/1557988319835985.

Lull, Cristina, Harry J. Wichers, and Huub F. J. Savelkoul. "Anti-inflammatory and Immunomodulating Properties of Fungal Metabolites." *Mediators of Inflammation* 2005:2 (June 9, 2005), 63–80. doi:10.1155/MI.2005.63.

Luo, Hua, Chi Teng Vong, Hanbin Chen, Yan Gao, Peng Lyu, Ling Qiu, Mingming Zhao, et al. "Naturally Occurring Anticancer Compounds: Shining from Chinese Herbal Medicine." *Chinese Medicine* 14:48 (2019). doi:10.1186/s13020-019 -0270-9.

Lynn, Becky K., Julia D. López, Collin Miller, Judy Thompson, and E. Cristian Campian. "The Relationship between Marijuana Use Prior to Sex and Sexual Function in Women." *Sexual Medicine* 7:2 (June 1, 2019), 192–97. doi:10.1016/j .esxm.2019.01.003.

Ma, Xiuzhen, Junfeng Deng, Xinmu Cui, Qi Chen, and Weihua Wang. "Berberine Exhibits Antioxidative Effects and Reduces Apoptosis of the Vaginal Epithelium in Bacterial Vaginosis." *Experimental and Therapeutic Medicine* 18:3 (September 2019), 2122–30. doi:10.3892/etm.2019.7772.

Mahboubi, Mohaddese, and Mona Mahboubi. "Hepatoprotection by Dandelion *(Taraxacum officinale)* and Mechanisms." *Asian Pacific Journal of Tropical Biomedicine* 10:1 (2020), 1–10. doi:10.4103/2221-1691.273081.

Malviya, Neelesh, Sanjay Jain, Vipin Bihari Gupta, and Savita Vyas. "Recent Studies on Aphrodisiac Herbs for the Management of Male Sexual Dysfunction—a Review." *Acta Poloniae Pharmaceutica* 68:1 (January–February 2011), 3–8. https://tinyurl.com/ux4cvy33.

Mares, Waleed Abid Al-Kadir, and Wisam S. Najam. "The Effect of Ginger on Semen Parameters and Serum FSH, LH & Testosterone of Infertile Men." *Medical Journal of Tikrit University* 18:182 (2012), 322–29. https://tinyurl .com/5y5vxnhb.

Martin, Sean A., Evan Atlantis, Kylie Lange, Anne W. Taylor, Peter O'Loughlin, and Gary A. Wittert. "Predictors of Sexual Dysfunction Incidence and Remission in Men." *Journal of Sexual Medicine* 11:5 (May 1, 2014), 1136–47. doi:10.1111/jsm.12483.

Mashour, Nick H., George I. Lin, and William H. Frishman. "Herbal Medicine for the Treatment of Cardiovascular Disease." *Archives of Internal Medicine* 158:20 (1998), 2225–34. doi:10.1001/archinte.158.20.2225.

McGovern, Patrick E., Armen Mirzoian, and Gretchen R. Hall. "Ancient Egyptian Herbal Wines." *Proceedings of the National Academy of Sciences* 106:18 (May 5, 2009), 7361–66. doi:10.1073/pnas.0811578106.

Meena, Jairam, Rakesh Ojha, A. V. Muruganandam, and Sairam Krishnamurthy. "*Asparagus racemosus* Competitively Inhibits In Vitro the Acetylcholine and

Monoamine Metabolizing Enzymes." *Neuroscience Letters* 503:1 (September 26, 2011), 6–9. doi:10.1016/j.neulet.2011.07.051.

Mehrandish, Reza, Aliasghar Rahimian, and Alireza Shahriary. "Heavy Metals Detoxification: A Review of Herbal Compounds for Chelation Therapy in Heavy Metals Toxicity." *Journal of Herbmed Pharmacology* 8:2 (2019), 69–77. doi:10.15171/jhp.2019.12.

Meissner, H. O., W. Kapczynski, A. Mscisz, and J. Lutomski. "Use of Gelatinized Maca *(Lepidium peruvianum)* in Early Postmenopausal Women." *International Journal of Biomedical Science* 1:1 (June 2005), 33–45. https://tinyurl.com/tpx38pah.

Mengs, Ulrich, Ralf-Torsten Pohl, and Todd Mitchell. "The Antidote of Choice in Patients with Acute Hepatotoxicity from Amatoxin Poisoning." *Current Pharmaceutical Biotechnology* 13:10 (August 2012), 1964–70. doi:10.2174/138920112802273353.

Microbicide Trials Network. "Cell Damage Caused by Use of Certain Personal Lubricants Does Not Increase HIV Risk, Lab Study Finds." *Science Daily,* November 7, 2012. https://tinyurl.com/pataabam.

Mink, Pamela J., Carolyn G. Scrafford, Leila M. Barraj, Lisa Harnack, Ching-Ping Hong, Jennifer A. Nettleton, and David R. Jacobs Jr. "Flavonoid Intake and Cardiovascular Disease Mortality: A Prospective Study in Postmenopausal Women." *American Journal of Clinical Nutrition* 85:3 (March 2007), 895–909. doi:10.1093/ajcn/85.3.895.

Mohammadi, Forouzan, Hossein Nikzad, Aliakbar Taherian, Javad Amini Mahabadi, and Mahdi Salehi. "Effects of Herbal Medicine on Male Infertility." *Anatomical Sciences Journal* 10:4 (November 2013). https://tinyurl.com/y26mycue.

Momoeda, Mikio, Hidetaka Sasaki, Eiko Tagashira, Masayuki Ogishima, Yuichi Takano, and Kazunori Ochiai. "Efficacy and Safety of *Vitex agnus-castus* Extract for Treatment of Premenstrual Syndrome in Japanese Patients: A Prospective, Open-Label Study." *Advances in Therapy* 31:3 (March 2014), 362–73. doi:10.1007/s12325-014-0106-z.

Murphy, Patricia A., Steven E. Kern, Frank Z. Stanczyk, and Carolyn L. Westhoff. "Interaction of St. John's Wort with Oral Contraceptives: Effects on the Pharmacokinetics of Norethindrone and Ethinyl Estradiol, Ovarian Activity and Breakthrough Bleeding." *Contraception* 71:6 (June 2005), 402–8. doi:10.1016/j.contraception.2004.11.004.

Nagel, Glen. "Mastering Menstruums in Herbal Extracts." Traditional Roots Conference, Portland, OR, 2017. https://tinyurl.com/2f9kbs3h.

Nair, Rajesh, Senthy Sellaturay, and Seshadri Sriprasad. "The History of Ginseng in the Management of Erectile Dysfunction in Ancient China (3500–2600 BCE)." *Indian Journal of Urology* 28:1 (January 2012), 15–20. doi:10.4103/0970-1591.94946.

Naseri, Rozita, Vahid Farnia, Katayoun Yazdchi, Mostafa Alikhani, Behrad Basanj, and Safora Salemi. "Comparison of *Vitex agnus-castus* Extracts with Placebo in Reducing Menopausal Symptoms: A Randomized Double-Blind Study." *Korean Journal of Family Medicine* 40:6 (November 2019), 362–67. doi:10.4082/kjfm.18.0067.

National Center for Complementary and Integrative Health. "Herb-Drug Interactions." *NCCIH Clinical Digest,* September 2015. https://tinyurl.com/skamjkb2.

National Institute of Diabetes and Digestive and Kidney Diseases. "Estrogens and Oral Contraceptives." In *LiverTox: Clinical and Research Information on Drug-Induced Liver Injury.* May 28, 2020. https://tinyurl.com/36xw6cvd.

Native American Ethnobotany DB. S.v. "taraxacum officinal." https://tinyurl.com/5bcndett.

Nguyen, Christopher, Ali Mehaidli, Kiruthika Baskaran, Sahibjot Grewal, Alaina Pupulin, Ivan Ruvinov, Benjamin Scaria, Krishan Parashar, Caleb Vegh, and Siyaram Pandey. "Dandelion Root and Lemongrass Extracts Induce Apoptosis, Enhance Chemotherapeutic Efficacy, and Reduce Tumour Xenograft Growth In Vivo in Prostate Cancer." *Complementary and Alternative Medicine* 2019:2951428. doi:10.1155/2019/2951428.

Nynas, Johnna, Puneet Narang, Murali K. Kolikonda, and Steven Lippmann. "Depression and Anxiety Following Early Pregnancy Loss: Recommendations for Primary Care Providers." *Primary Care Companion to CNS Disorders* 17:1 (2015). doi:10.4088/PCC.14r01721.

Olvera, María del Carmen Ramírez. "Composition of Plant Extracts That Increase Döderlein Bacilli, Used for the Treatment of Sexually Transmitted Diseases (STD) and the Human Papillomavirus (HPV), Having an Aphrodisiac Effect." Patent by María del Carmen Ramírez Olvera. Filed October 11, 2016. Application granted August 6, 2018. https://tinyurl.com/7p33t7am.

Ozgoli, Giti, Marjan Goli, and Fariborz Moattar. "Comparison of Effects of Ginger, Mefenamic Acid, and Ibuprofen on Pain in Women with Primary Dysmenorrhea." *Journal of Alternative and Complementary Medicine* 15:2 (February 2009), 129–32. doi:10.1089/acm.2008.0311.

Pacheco, Lara. "Oats *(Avena sativa)*." HerbRally, n.d. www.herbrally.com/monographs/oats.

Pamphlett, Roger, Laveniya Satgunaseelan, Stephen Kum Jew, Philip A. Doble, and David P. Bishop. "Elemental Bioimaging Shows Mercury and Other Toxic Metals in Normal Breast Tissue and in Breast Cancers." *PloS One,* January 31, 2020. doi:10.1371/journal.pone.0228226.

Park, Chan Jin, Radwa Barakat, Alexander Ulanov, Zhong Li, Po-Ching Lin, Karen Chiu, Sherry Zhou, et al. "Sanitary Pads and Diapers Contain Higher Phthalate Contents Than Those in Common Commercial Plastic Products." *Reproductive Toxicology* 84 (March 2019), 114–21. doi:10.1016/j.reprotox.2019.01.005.

Pazhohideh, Zahra, Solmaz Mohammadi, Nosrat Bahrami, Faraz Mojab, Parvin Abedi, and Elham Maraghi. "The Effect of *Calendula officinalis* versus Metronidazole on Bacterial Vaginosis in Women: A Double-Blind Randomized Controlled Trial." *Journal of Advanced Pharmaceutical Technology & Research* 9:1 (January–March 2018), 15–19. doi:10.4103/japtr.JAPTR_305_17.

Peters, Ember. "Wild Carrot Monograph." *Wild Current Herbalism,* December 2014.

Petrovska, Biljana Bauer. "Historical Review of Medicinal Plants' Usage." *Pharmacognosy Reviews* 6:11 (January 2012), 1–5. doi:10.4103/0973-7847.95849.

Pivonello, Claudia, Giovanna Muscogiuri, Antonio Nardone, Francesco Garifalos, Donatella Paola Provvisiero, Nunzia Verde, Cristina de Angelis, et al. "Bisphenol A: An Emerging Threat to Female Fertility." *Reproductive Biology and Endocrinology* 18:22 (2020). doi:10.1186/s12958-019-0558-8.

Potroz, Michael G., and Nam-Joon Cho. "Natural Products for the Treatment of Trachoma and *Chlamydia trachomatis*." *Molecules* 20:3 (March 2015), 4180–203. doi:10.3390/molecules20034180.

Powles, Trevor J., Anthony Howell, D. Gareth Evans, Eugene V. McCloskey, Sue Ashley, Rosemary Greenhalgh, Jenny Affen, Lesley Ann Flook, and Alwynne Tidy. "Red Clover Isoflavones Are Safe and Well Tolerated in Women with a Family History of Breast Cancer." *Journal of the British Menopause Society* 14:1 (March 2008), 6–12. doi:10.1258/mi.2007.007033.

Rahmani, Yousef, Khadijeh Chaleh, Afshar Shahmohammadi, and Shahla Safari. "Effect of Herbal Medicine on Vaginal Epithelial Cells: A Systematic Review and Meta-Analysis." *Journal of Menopausal Medicine* 24:1 (April 2018), 11–16. doi:10.6118/jmm.2018.24.1.11.

Riddle, John M., and J. Worth Estes. "Oral Contraceptives in Ancient and Medieval Times." *American Scientist* 80:3 (May 1992). doi:10.2307/29774642.

Rier, Sherry, and Warren G. Foster. "Environmental Dioxins and Endometriosis." *Toxicological Sciences* 70:2 (December 2002), 161–70. doi:10.1093/toxsci/70.2.161.

Rotem, Carmela, and Boris Kaplan. "Phyto-Female Complex for the Relief of Hot Flushes, Night Sweats and Quality of Sleep: Randomized, Controlled, Double-Blind Pilot Study." *Gynecological Endocrinology* 23:2 (February 2007), 117–22. doi:10.1080/09513590701200900.

Rubin, Lee Hullender, Dara Cantor, and Benjamin L. Marx. "Recurrent Pregnancy Loss and Traditional Chinese Medicine." *Medical Acupuncture* 25:3 (June 2013), 232–37. doi:10.1089/acu.2012.0911.

Saffari, Elnaz, Sakineh Mohammad-Alizadeh-Charandabi, Mohammad Adibpour, Mojgan Mirghafourvand, and Yousef Javadzadeh. "Comparing the Effects of *Calendula officinalis* and Clotrimazole on Vaginal Candidiasis: A Randomized Controlled Trial." *Women and Health* 57:10 (November–December 2017), 1145–60. doi:10.1080/03630242.2016.1263272.

Safron, Adam. "What Is Orgasm? A Model of Sexual Trance and Climax Via Rhythmic Entrainment." *Socioaffective Neuroscience and Psychology* 6 (October 25, 2016). doi:10.3402/snp.v6.31763.

Saxena, Ram Chandra, Rakesh Singh, Parveen Kumar, Mahendra P. Singh Negi, Vinod S. Saxena, Periasamy Geetharani, Joseph Joshua Allan, and Kudiganti Venkateshwarlu. "Efficacy of an Extract of *Ocimum tenuiflorum* (OciBest) in the Management of General Stress: A Double-Blind, Placebo-Controlled Study." *Complementary and Alternative Medicine* 2012:894509. doi:10.1155/2012/894509.

Scholey, Andrew B., Stephen J. French, Penelope J. Morris, David O. Kennedy, Anthea L. Milne, and Crystal F. Haskell. "Consumption of Cocoa Flavanols Results in Acute Improvements in Mood and Cognitive Performance during Sustained Mental Effort." *Journal of Psychopharmacology* 24:10 (October 2010), 1505–14. doi:10.1177/0269881109106923.

Science Direct. "Astragalus." 2018. https://tinyurl.com/3tuddpt2.

Shankar, G. S. "Serotonin and Sexual Dysfunction." *Journal of Autacoids and Hormones* 5 (2015), e129. doi:10.4172/2161-0479.1000e129.

Shin, Byung-Cheul, Myeong Soo Lee, Eun Jin Yang, Hyun-Suk Lim, and Edzard Ernst. "Maca *(L. meyenii)* for Improving Sexual Function: A Systematic Review." *BMC Complementary and Alternative Medicine* 2010:10, 44. doi:10.1186/1472-6882-10-44.

Sigler, Kara. "TransNatural for Professionals." American Herbalists Guild, n.d. https://tinyurl.com/226ty87u.

Simsa, Peter, Attila Mihalyi, Greet Schoeters, Gudrun Koppen, Cleophas M. Kyama, Elly M. Den Hond, Vilmos Fülöp, and Thomas M. D'Hooghe.

"Increased Exposure to Dioxin-like Compounds Is Associated with Endometriosis in a Case-Control Study in Women." *Reproductive Biomedicine Online* 20 (2010), 681–88. doi:10.1016/j.rbmo.2010.01.018. https://tinyurl.com/rj7n9u3n.

Skovlund, Charlotte Wessel, Lina Steinrud Mørch, Lars Vedel Kessing, and Øjvind Lidegaard. "Association of Hormonal Contraception with Depression." *JAMA Psychiatry* 73:11 (November 2016), 1154–62. doi:10.1001/jamapsychiatry.2016.2387.

Smith, Brandi Patrice, and Zeynep Madak-Erdogan. "Urban Neighborhood and Residential Factors Associated with Breast Cancer in African American Women: A Systematic Review." *Hormones and Cancer* 9 (2018), 71–81. doi:10.1007/s12672-018-0325-x.

Sprinkle, Annie, and Beth Stephens. "Ecosexuality: The Story of Our Love with the Earth." In *Assuming the Ecosexual Position: The Earth as Lover.* Chicago: University of Chicago Press, 2021.

Stansbury, Jillian. "Botanical Influences on Metabolic Syndrome." Presentation. American Herbalists Guild, n.d. https://tinyurl.com/nup7cffk.

Stansbury, Jillian. "Melissa and Other Dopaminergic Herbs Useful in Treatment of PCOS." *Naturopathic Doctor News and Review,* August 6, 2009. https://tinyurl.com/rzpk5xy.

Stobart, Anne. "The Working of Herbs, Part 5: Medicinal Herb Constituents and Actions." The Recipes Project, January 7, 2014. https://recipes.hypotheses.org/3076.

Sweet, Victoria. "Hildegard of Bingen and the Greening of Medieval Medicine." *Bulletin of the History of Medicine* 73:3 (Fall 1999), 381–403. doi:10.1353/bhm.1999.0140.

Tassell, Mary C., Rosari Kingston, Deirdre Gilroy, Mary Lehane, and Ambrose Furey. "Hawthorn (*Crataegus* spp.) in the Treatment of Cardiovascular Disease." *Pharmacognosy Reviews* 4:7 (January–June 2010), 32–41. doi:10.4103/0973-7847.65324.

Teas, Jane, Sylvia Vena, D. Lindsie Cone, and Mohammad Irhimeh. "The Consumption of Seaweed as a Protective Factor in the Etiology of Breast Cancer: Proof of Principle." *Journal of Applied Phycology* 25:3 (2013), 771–79. doi:10.1007/s10811-012-9931-0.

Tseng, Ying-Fen, Chung-Hey Chen, and Yi-Hsin Yang. "Rose Tea for Relief of Primary Dysmenorrhea in Adolescents: A Randomized Controlled Trial in Taiwan." *Journal of Midwifery & Women's Health* 50:5 (September–October 2005), e51–57. doi:10.1016/j.jmwh.2005.06.003.

U.S. Centers for Disease Control and Prevention. "*Health, United States* Spotlight: Racial and Ethnic Disparities in Heart Disease." April 2019. https://tinyurl.com/4p2zx68t.

Vallée, Alexandre, and Yves Lecarpentier. "Curcumin and Endometriosis." *International Journal of Molecular Sciences* 21:7 (April 2020), 2440. doi:10.3390/ijms21072440.

Van Die, Margaret Diana, Henry G. Burger, Helena J. Teede, and Kerry M. Bone. "*Vitex agnus-castus* (Chaste-Tree/Berry) in the Treatment of Menopause-Related Complaints." *Journal of Alternative and Complementary Medicine* 15:8 (August 2009), 853–62. doi:10.1089/acm.2008.0447.

Vidyashankar, Satyakumar, O. S. Thiyagarajan, R. Sandeep Varma, L. M. Sharath Kumar, Uddagiri Venkanna Babu, and Pralhad Sadashiv Patki. "Ashwagandha *(Withania somnifera)* Supercritical CO_2 Extract Derived Withanolides Mitigates Bisphenol A Induced Mitochondrial Toxicity in HepG2 Cells." *Toxicology Reports* (Ireland) 1 (July 4, 2014), 1004–12. doi:10.1016/j.toxrep.2014.06.008.

Vynograd, N., I. Vynograd, and Z. Sosnowski. "A Comparative Multi-Centre Study of the Efficacy of Propolis, Acyclovir and Placebo in the Treatment of Genital Herpes (HSV)." *Phytomedicine* 7:1 (March 2000), 1–6. doi:10.1016/S0944-7113(00)80014-8.

Wallenfeldt, Jeff. "Salem Witch Trials: History & Causes." *Encyclopedia Britannica,* n.d. www.britannica.com/event/Salem-witch-trials.

Wang, Tong, Bing Xue, Hui Shao, Shu-Yu Wang, Li Bai, Cheng-Hong Yin, Huan-Ying Zhao, et al. "Effect of Dandelion Extracts on the Proliferation of Ovarian Granulosa Cells and Expression of Hormone Receptors." *Chinese Medical Journal* 131:14 (July 20, 2018), 1694–1701. doi:10.4103/0366-6999.235864.

Westphal, Lynn M., Mary Lake Polan, Aileen Sontag Trant, and Stephen B. Mooney. "A Nutritional Supplement for Improving Fertility in Women: A Pilot Study." *Journal of Reproductive Medicine* 49:4 (April 2004), 289–93. https://tinyurl.com/p34vaf54.

Whitecoat Strategies. "Premenstrual Breast Pain Is Reduced with Red Clover Supplement." Whitecoat Strategies, Washington, DC, November 15, 2001. https://tinyurl.com/xpecejv7.

Whorton, James C. "Cultism to CAM: The Flexner Report Reconsidered." *Complementary Health Practice Review* 6:2 (Winter–Spring 2001).

Williamson, Elizabeth, Samuel Driver, and Karen Baxter, eds. *Stockley's Herbal Medicines Interactions.* Chicago: Pharmaceutical Press, 2009. https://tinyurl.com/2tcnukwp.

Wink, Michael. "Modes of Action of Herbal Medicines and Plant Secondary Metabolites." *Medicines (Basel)* 2:3 (September 1, 2015), 251–86. doi:10.3390/medicines2030251.

Women's Voices for the Earth. "Always Pads Testing Results." n.d. https://tinyurl .com/4wuvsapc.

Wong, Rachel H. X., Peter R. C. Howe, Janet Bryan, Alison M. Coates, Jonathan D. Buckley, and Narelle M. Berry. "Chronic Effects of a Wild Green Oat Extract Supplementation on Cognitive Performance in Older Adults: A Randomised, Double-Blind, Placebo-Controlled, Crossover Trial." *Nutrients* 4:5 (May 1, 2012), 331–42. doi:10.3390/nu4050331.

Wu, Meng-Hsing, Pei-Fang Su, Wei-Ying Chu, New Geok Huey, Chih-Wei Lin, Huang-Tz Ou, and Chung-Ying Lin. "Quality of Life and Pregnancy Outcomes among Women Undergoing In Vitro Fertilization Treatment: A Longitudinal Cohort Study." *Journal of the Formosan Medical Association* 119:1 (January 2020), 471–79. doi:10.1016/j.jfma.2019.06.015.

Wu, Meng-Hsing, Pei-Fang Su, Wei-Ying Chu, Chih-Wei Lin, New Geok Huey, Chung-Ying Lin, and Huang-Tz Ou. "Quality of Life among Infertile Women with Endometriosis Undergoing IVF Treatment and Their Pregnancy Out-comes." *Journal of Psychosomatic Obstetrics & Gynecology* 42:1 (2021). doi:10.1080 /0167482X.2020.1758659.

Xi, Sisi, Eckehard Liske, Shuyu Wang, Jianli Liu, Zhonglan Zhang, Li Geng, Lina Hu, et al. "Effect of Isopropanolic *Cimicifuga racemosa* Extract on Uterine Fibroids in Comparison with Tibolone among Patients of a Recent Ran-domized, Double Blind, Parallel-Controlled Study in Chinese Women with Menopausal Symptoms." *Complementary and Alternative Medicine* 2014:717686. doi:10.1155/2014/717686.

Xiao, An, Hai-Ying He, Qing Chen, and Shi-Wu Ma. "Drug-Induced Liver Injury Due to *Lepidium meyenii* (Maca) Medicinal Liquor." *Chinese Medical Journal* 130:24 (December 20, 2017), 3005–6. doi:10.4103/0366-6999.220314.

Yarnell, Eric. "Herbs Against Human Papillomavirus." *Alternative and Complemen-tary Therapies* 21:2 (April 2015), 71–76. doi:10.1089/act.2015.21205.

Yildirim, Ayse, Gulay Gulbol Duran, Nizami Duran, Kemal Jenedi, Behiye Sezgin Bolgul, Meral Miraloglu, and Mustafa Muz. "Antiviral Activity of Hatay Prop-olis Against Replication of Herpes Simplex Virus Type 1 and Type 2." *Medical Science Monitor* 22 (2016), 422–30. doi:10.12659/MSM.897282.

Youssef, Dima A., Alan N. Peiris, Jim L. Kelley, and William B. Grant. "The Possible Roles of Vitamin D and Curcumin in Treating Gonorrhea." *Medical Hypotheses* 81:1 (July 2013), 131–35. doi:10.1016/j.mehy.2013.04.013.

Zhang, Jing-Shu, Zhao-Huan Guia, Zhi-Yong Zou, Bo-Yi Yang, Jun Ma, Jin Jing, Hai-Jun Wang, et al. "Long-term Exposure to Ambient Air Pollution and Metabolic Syndrome in Children and Adolescents: A National Cross-sectional Study in China." *Environment International* 148 (March 2021). doi:10.1016/j.envint.2021.106383.

Zhao, Hong, Qingyuan Zhang, Ling Zhao, Xu Huang, Jincai Wang, and Xinmei Kang. "Spore Powder of *Ganoderma lucidum* Improves Cancer-Related Fatigue in Breast Cancer Patients Undergoing Endocrine Therapy: A Pilot Clinical Trial." *Complementary and Alternative Medicine* 2012:809614. doi:10.1155/2012/809614.

Zheng, Weilin, Lixing Cao, Zheng Xu, Yuanyuan Ma, and Xuefang Liang. "Anti-Angiogenic Alternative and Complementary Medicines for the Treatment of Endometriosis: A Review of Potential Molecular Mechanisms." *Complementary and Alternative Medicine* 2018:4128984. doi:10.1155/2018/4128984.

Zhi, Xu, Ken-Ichi Honda, Koji Ozaki, Takuya Misugi, Toshiyuki Sumi, and Osamu Ishiko. "Dandelion T-1 Extract Up-Regulates Reproductive Hormone Receptor Expression in Mice." *International Journal of Molecular Medicine* 20:3 (September 2007), 287–92. https://pubmed.ncbi.nlm.nih.gov/17671731.

Index

Acknowledgments

To my early mentors and teachers in the herbal realm: Sandie, Caroline, Natacha, and Danièle. Thank you for introducing me to the wisdom of plants.

Thanks to my dear friends and family Robert, Jay, Clo, Isabelle, Ronald, Léon, and Andrée.

Thanks to my neighbors and friends Tricia, Michael, Atma (and the others who circle near us on the island) for the inspiration and for giving me regular opportunities to *not* write.

Thank you to my colleagues and friends Dionne and Becky for the encouragement and support and for beta-reading.

Thank you to my research assistant, Shelby D. Gibson, who offered valuable ongoing help and support.

Thanks to my editor, Shayna Keyles, and the whole team at North Atlantic Books, who offered steadfast support and encouragement—I couldn't have dreamed of a better team to work with.

A heartfelt thanks to you, dear reader, for joining me on this journey of healing and reclamation of our pleasure, health, and agency.

And finally, thank you to my husband and partner in herbs and life, Kevin, for being an unending source of inspiration and support in every way.

About the Author

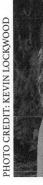

MARIE WHITE is an herbalist and author. She has published extensively on the topic of medicinal herbs, nature connection, and well-being. Originally from Montreal, Marie now calls the West Coast home. She tends medicinal herb gardens, writes, teaches, hosts herbal events, and finds creative ways to work with herbs as a gateway for advocacy, pleasure, and liberation.

Marie offers workshops and courses both online and in person. Her writing has appeared in multiple magazines, blogs, and popular online herbal education. She offers intimate herbal retreats and one-on-one consultations to foster sexual, reproductive, and hormonal health with medicinal herbs. Marie trains other herbalists and natural-health practitioners in the intimate herbalism method so they may better serve their clients with the help of tried-and-true herbal protocols and practice.

About North Atlantic Books

North Atlantic Books (NAB) is a 501(c)(3) nonprofit publisher committed to a bold exploration of the relationships between mind, body, spirit, culture, and nature. Founded in 1974, NAB aims to nurture a holistic view of the arts, sciences, humanities, and healing. To make a donation or to learn more about our books, authors, events, and newsletter, please visit www.northatlanticbooks.com.